A
GUIDE
TO
HOSPITALS
AND NURSING

A Collection of
Writings and Excerpts.

By

FLORENCE NIGHTINGALE

WITH AN
INTRODUCTORY CHAPTER
BY LYTTON STRACHEY

"Lo! in that house of misery,
A lady with a lamp I see,
Pass through the glimmering gloom,
And flit from room to room."

LONGFELLOW.

CONTENTS

FLORENCE NIGHTINGALE

By Lytton Strachey

I

Every one knows the popular conception of Florence Nightingale. The saintly, self-sacrificing woman, the delicate maiden of high degree who threw aside the pleasures of a life of ease to succour the afflicted, the Lady with the Lamp, gliding through the horrors of the hospital at Scutari, and consecrating with the radiance of her goodness the dying soldier's couch—the vision is familiar to all. But the truth was different. The Miss Nightingale of fact was not as facile fancy painted her. She worked in another fashion, and towards another end; she moved under the stress of an impetus which finds no place in the popular imagination. A Demon possessed her. Now demons, whatever else they may be, are full of interest. And so it happens that in the real Miss Nightingale there was more that was interesting than in the legendary one; there was also less that was agreeable.

Her family was extremely well-to-do, and connected by marriage with a spreading circle of other well-to-do families. There was a large country house in Derbyshire; there was another in the New Forest; there were Mayfair rooms for the London season and all its finest parties; there were tours on the Continent with even more than the usual number of Italian operas and of glimpses at the celebrities of Paris. Brought up among such advantages, it was only natural to suppose that

Florence would show a proper appreciation of them by doing her duty in that state of life unto which it had pleased God to call her—in other words, by marrying, after a fitting number of dances and dinner-parties, an eligible gentleman, and living happily ever afterwards. Her sister, her cousins, all the young ladies of her acquaintance, were either getting ready to do this or had already done it. It was inconceivable that Florence should dream of anything else; yet dream she did. Ah! To do her duty in that state of life unto which it had pleased God to call her! Assuredly she would not be behindhand in doing her duty; but unto what state of life *had* it pleased God to call her? That was the question. God's calls are many, and they are strange. Unto what state of life had it pleased Him to call Charlotte Corday, or Elizabeth of Hungary? What was that secret voice in her ear, if it was not a call? Why had she felt, from her earliest years, those mysterious promptings towards . . . she hardly knew what, but certainly towards something very different from anything around her? Why, as a child in the nursery, when her sister had shown a healthy pleasure in tearing her dolls to pieces, had *she* shown an almost morbid one in sewing them up again? Why was she driven now to minister to the poor in their cottages, to watch by sick-beds, to put her dog's wounded paw into elaborate splints as if it was a human being? Why was her head filled with queer imaginations of the country house at Embley turned, by some enchantment, into a hospital, with herself as matron moving about among the beds? Why was even her vision of heaven itself filled with suffering patients to whom she was being useful? So she dreamed and wondered, and, taking out her diary, she poured into it the agitations of her soul. And then the bell rang, and it was time to go and dress for dinner.

As the years passed, a restlessness began to grow upon her. She was unhappy, and at last she knew it. Mrs. Nightingale, too, began to notice that there was something wrong. It was very odd; what could be the matter with dear Flo? Mr. Nightingale suggested that a husband might be advisable; but the curious

8

thing was that she seemed to take no interest in husbands. And with her attractions, and her accomplishments, too I There was nothing in the world to prevent her making a really brilliant match. But no! She would think of nothing but how to satisfy that singular craving of hers to be *doing* something. As if there was not plenty to do in any case, in the ordinary way, at home. There was the china to look after, and there was her father to be read to after dinner. Mrs. Nightingale could not understand it; and then one day her perplexity was changed to consternation and alarm. Florence announced an extreme desire to go to Salisbury Hospital for several months as a nurse; and she confessed to some visionary plan of eventually setting up in a house of her own in a neighbouring village, and there founding "something like a Protestant Sisterhood, without vows, for women of educated feelings." The whole scheme was summarily brushed aside as preposterous; and Mrs. Nightingale, after the first shock of terror, was able to settle down again more or less comfortably to her embroidery. But Florence, who was now twenty-five and felt that the dream of her life had been shattered, came near to desperation.

And, indeed, the difficulties in her path were great. For not only was it an almost unimaginable thing in those days for a woman of means to make her own way in the world and to live in independence, but the particular profession for which Florence was clearly marked out both by her instincts and her capacities was at that time a peculiarly disreputable one. A "nurse" meant then a coarse old woman, always ignorant, usually dirty, often brutal, a Mrs. Gamp, in bunched-up sordid garments, tippling at the brandy-bottle or indulging in worse irregularities. The nurses in the hospitals were especially notorious for immoral conduct; sobriety was almost unknown among them; and they could hardly be trusted to carry out the simplest medical duties. Certainly, things have changed since those days; and that they *have* changed is due, far more than to any other human being, to Miss Nightingale herself. It is not to be wondered at that her parents should have shuddered at the notion of their daughter devoting her life to such an occupation. "It was as if," she herself said afterwards, "I had wanted to be a kitchen-maid." Yet the want, absurd, impracticable as it was, not only remained fixed immovably in her heart, but grew in intensity day by day. Her wretchedness deepened into a morbid melancholy. Everything about her was vile, and she herself, it was clear, to have deserved such misery, was even viler than her surroundings. Yes, she had sinned—"standing before God's judgment seat." "No one," she declared, "has so grieved the Holy Spirit"; of that she was quite certain. It was in vain that she prayed to be delivered from vanity and hypocrisy, and she could not bear to smile or to be gay, "because she hated God to hear her laugh, as if she had not repented of her sin."

A weaker spirit would have been overwhelmed by the load of such distresses—would have yielded or snapped. But this extraordinary young woman held firm, and fought her way to victory. With an amazing persistency, during the eight years that followed her rebuff over Salisbury Hospital, she struggled and worked and planned. While superficially she was carrying on the life of a brilliant girl in high society, while internally she was a prey to the tortures of regret and of remorse, she yet possessed the energy to collect the knowledge and to undergo the experience which alone could enable her to do what she had determined she would do in the end. In secret she devoured the reports of medical commissions, the pamphlets of sanitary authorities, the histories of hospitals and homes. She spent the intervals of the London season in ragged schools and workhouses. When she went abroad with her family, she used her spare time so well that there was hardly a great hospital in Europe with which she was not acquainted, hardly a great city whose slums she had not passed through. She managed to spend some days in a convent school in Rome, and some weeks as a "Sœur de Charité" in Paris.

Then, while her mother and sister were taking the waters at Carlsbad, she succeeded in slipping off to a nursing institution at Kaiserswerth, where she remained for more than three months. This was the critical event of her life. The experience which she gained as a nurse at Kaiserswerth formed the foundation of all her future action and finally fixed her in her career.

But one other trial awaited her. The allurements of the world she had brushed aside with disdain and loathing; she had resisted the subtler temptation which, in her weariness, had sometimes come upon her, of devoting her baffled energies to art or literature; the last ordeal appeared in the shape of a desirable young man. Hitherto, her lovers had been nothing to her but an added burden and a mockery; but now——. For a moment, she wavered. A new feeling swept over her—a feeling which she had never known before, which she was never to know again. The most powerful and the profoundest of all the instincts of humanity laid claim upon her. But it rose before her, that instinct, arrayed—how could it be otherwise?—in the inevitable habiliments of a Victorian marriage; and she had the strength to stamp it underfoot. "I have an intellectual nature which requires satisfaction," she noted, "and that would find it in him. I have a passional nature which requires satisfaction, and that would find it in him. I have a moral, an active nature which requires satisfaction, and that would not find it in his life. Sometimes I think that I will satisfy my passional nature at all events. ..." But no, she knew in her heart that it could not be. "To be nailed to a continuation and exaggeration of my present life ... to put it out of my power ever to be able to seize the chance of forming for myself a true and rich life"—that would be a suicide. She made her choice, and refused what was at least a certain happiness for a visionary good which might never come to her at all. And so she returned to her old life of waiting and bitterness. "The thoughts and feelings that I have now," she wrote, "I can remember since I was six years old. A profession, a trade, a necessary occupation, something to fill and employ all my faculties, I have always felt essential to me, I have always longed for. The first thought I can remember, and the last, was nursing work; and in the absence of this, education work, but more the education of the bad than of the young. ... Everything has been tried, foreign travel, kind friends, everything. My God! What is to become of me?" A desirable young man? Dust and ashes I What was there desirable in such a thing as that? "In my thirty-first year," she noted in her diary, "I see nothing desirable but death."

Three more years passed, and then at last the pressure of time told; her family seemed to realise that she was old enough and strong enough to have her way; and she became the superintendent of a charitable nursing home in Harley Street. She had gained her independence, though it was in a meagre sphere enough; and her mother was still not quite resigned: surely Florence might at least spend the summer in the country. At times, indeed, among her intimates, Mrs. Nightingale almost wept. "We are ducks," she said with tears in her eyes, "who have hatched a wild swan." But the poor lady was wrong; it was not a swan that they had hatched; it was an eagle.

II

Miss Nightingale had been a year in her nursing-home in Harley Street, when Fate knocked at the door. The Crimean War broke out; the battle of the Alma was fought; and the terrible condition of our military hospitals at Scutari began to be known in England. It sometimes happens that the plans of Providence are a little difficult to follow, but on this occasion all was plain; there was a perfect co-ordination of events. For years Miss Nightingale had been getting ready; at last she was prepared—experienced, free, mature, yet still young—she was thirty-four—desirous to serve, accustomed to command: at that precise moment the desperate need of a great nation came, and she was there to satisfy it. If the war had fallen a few years earlier, she would have lacked the knowledge, perhaps even the power, for such a work; a few years later and she would, no doubt, have been fixed in the routine of some absorbing task, and moreover, she would have been growing old. Nor was it only the coincidence of Time that was remarkable. It so fell out that Sidney Herbert was at the War Office and in the Cabinet; and Sidney Herbert was an intimate friend of Miss Nightingale's, convinced, from personal experience in charitable work, of her supreme capacity. After such premises, it seems hardly more than a matter of course that her letter, in which she offered her services for the East, and Sidney Herbert's letter, in which he asked for them, should actually have crossed in the post. Thus it all happened, without a hitch. The appointment was made, and even Mrs. Nightingale, overawed by the magnitude of the venture, could only approve. A pair of faithful friends offered themselves as personal attendants; thirty-eight nurses were collected; and within a week of the crossing of the letters Miss Nightingale, amid a great burst of popular enthusiasm, left for Constantinople.

Among the numerous letters which she received on her departure was one from Dr. Manning, who at that time was working in comparative obscurity as a Catholic priest in Bayswater. "God will keep you," he wrote, "and my prayer for you will be that your one object of Worship, Pattern of Imitation, and source of consolation and strength may be the Sacred Heart of our Divine Lord."

To what extent Dr. Manning's prayer was answered must remain a matter of doubt; but this much is certain, that, if ever a prayer was needed, it was needed then for Florence Nightingale. For dark as had been the picture of the state of affairs at Scutari, revealed to the English public in the despatches of the *Times* correspondent and in a multitude of private letters, yet the reality turned out to be darker still. What had occurred was, in brief,

13

the complete break-down of our medical arrangements at the seat of war. The origins of this awful failure were complex and manifold; they stretched back through long years of peace and carelessness in England; they could be traced through endless ramifications of administrative incapacity—from the inherent faults of confused systems to the petty bunglings of minor officials, from the inevitable ignorance of Cabinet Ministers to the fatal exactitudes of narrow routine. In the inquiries which followed it was clearly shown that the evil was in reality that worst of all evils—one which has been caused by nothing in particular and for which no one in particular is to blame. The whole organisation of the war machine was incompetent and out of date. The old Duke had sat for a generation at the Horse Guards repressing innovations with an iron hand. There was an extraordinary overlapping of authorities, an almost incredible shifting of responsibilities to and fro. As for such a notion as the creation and the maintenance of a really adequate medical service for the army—in that atmosphere of aged chaos, how could it have entered anybody's head? Before the war, the easy-going officials at Westminster were naturally persuaded that all was well—or at least as well as could be expected; when some one, for instance, actually had the temerity to suggest the formation of a corps of army nurses, he was at once laughed out of court. When the war had begun, the gallant British officers in control of affairs had other things to think about than the petty details of medical organisation. Who had bothered with such trifles in the Peninsula? And surely, on that occasion, we had done pretty well. Thus the most obvious precautions were neglected, the most necessary preparations put off from day to day. The principal medical officer of the army, Dr. Hall, was summoned from India at a moment's notice, and was unable to visit England before taking up his duties at the front. And it was not until after the battle of the Alma, when we had been at war for many months, that we acquired hospital accommodation at

Scutari for more than a thousand men. Errors, follies, and vices on the part of individuals there doubtless were; but, in the general reckoning, they were of small account—insignificant symptoms of the deep disease of the body politic—the enormous calamity of administrative collapse.

Miss Nightingale arrived at Scutari—a suburb of Constantinople, on the Asiatic side of the Bosphorus—on November 4th, 1854; it was ten days after the battle of Balaclava, and the day before the battle of Inkerman. The organisation of the hospitals, which had already given way under the stress of the battle of the Alma, was now to be subjected to the further pressure which these two desperate and bloody engagements implied. Great detachments of wounded were already beginning to pour in. The men. after receiving such summary treatment as could be given them at the smaller hospitals in the Crimea itself, were forthwith shipped in batches of two hundred across the Black Sea to Scutari. This voyage was in normal times one of four days and a half; but the times were no longer normal, and now the transit often lasted for a fortnight or three weeks. It received, not without reason, the name of "the middle passage." Between, and sometimes on the decks, the wounded, the sick, and the dying were crowded—men who had just undergone the amputation of limbs, men in the clutches of fever or of frostbite, men in the last stages of dysentery and cholera—without beds, sometimes without blankets, often hardly clothed. The one or two surgeons on board did what they could; but medical stores were lacking, and the only form of nursing available was that provided by a handful of invalid soldiers, who were usually themselves prostrate by the end of the voyage. There was no other food beside the ordinary salt rations of ship diet; and even the water was sometimes so stored that it was out of reach of the weak. For many months, the average of deaths during these voyages was 74 in the thousand; the corpses were shot out into the waters; and who shall say that they were the most unfortunate? At Scutari, the landing-stage, constructed with all the perverseness of Oriental ingenuity, could only be approached with great difficulty, and, in rough weather, not at all. When it was reached, what remained of the men in the ships had first to be disembarked, and then conveyed up a steep slope of a quarter of a mile to the nearest of the hospitals. The most serious cases might be put upon stretchers—for there were far too few for all; the rest were carried or dragged up the hill by such convalescent soldiers as could be got together, who were not too obviously infirm for the work. At last the journey was accomplished; slowly, one by one, living or dying, the wounded were carried up into the hospital. And in the hospital what did they find?

Lasciate ogni speranza, voi ch'entrate: the delusive doors bore no such inscription; and yet behind them Hell yawned. Want, neglect, confusion, misery—in every shape and in every degree of intensity—filled the endless corridors and the vast apartments of the gigantic barrack-house, which, without forethought or preparation, had been hurriedly set aside as the chief shelter for the victims of the war. The very building itself was radically defective. Huge sewers underlay it, and cess-pools loaded with filth wafted their poison into the upper rooms. The floors were in so rotten a condition that many of them could not be scrubbed; the! walls were thick with dirt; incredible multitudes of vermin swarmed everywhere. And, enormous as the building was, it was yet too small. It contained four miles of beds, crushed together so close that there was but just room to pass between them. Under such conditions, the most elaborate system of ventilation might well have been at fault; but here there was no ventilation. The stench was indescribable. "I have been well acquainted," said Miss Nightingale, "with the dwellings of the worst parts of most of the great cities in Europe, but have never been in any atmosphere which I could compare with that of the Barrack Hospital at night." The structural defects were equalled by the deficiencies in the commonest objects of hospital use. There

16

were not enough bedsteads; the sheets were of canvas, and so coarse that the wounded men recoiled from them, begging to be left in their blankets; there was no bedroom furniture of any kind, and empty beer-bottles were used for candlesticks. There were no basins, no towels, no soap, no brooms, no mops, no trays, no plates; there were neither slippers nor scissors, neither shoe-brushes nor blacking; there were no knives or forks or spoons. The supply of fuel was constantly deficient. The cooking arrangements were preposterously inadequate, and the laundry was a farce. As for purely medical materials, the tale was no better. Stretchers, splints, bandages—all were lacking; and so were the most ordinary drugs.

To replace such wants, to struggle against such difficulties, there was a handful of men overburdened by the strain of ceaseless work, bound down by the traditions of official routine, and enfeebled either by old age or inexperience or sheer incompetence. They had proved utterly unequal to their task. The principal doctor was lost in the imbecilities of a senile optimism. The wretched official whose business it was to provide for the wants of the hospital was tied, fast hand and foot by red tape. A few of the younger doctors struggled valiantly, but what could they do? Unprepared, disorganised, with such help only as they could find among the miserable band of convalescent soldiers drafted off to tend their sick comrades, they were faced with disease, mutilation, and death in all their most appalling forms, crowded multitudinously about them in an ever increasing mass. They were like men in a shipwreck, fighting, not for safety, but for the next moment's bare existence—to gain, by yet another frenzied effort, some brief respite from the waters of destruction.

In these surroundings, those who had been long inured to scenes of human suffering—surgeons with a world-wide knowledge of agonies, soldiers familiar with fields of carnage, missionaries with remembrances of famine and of plague—yet found a depth of horror which they had never known before.

There were moments, there were places, in the Barrack Hospital at Scutari, where the strongest hand was struck with trembling, and the boldest eye would turn away its gaze.

Miss Nightingale came, and she, at any rate, in that Inferno, did not abandon hope. For one thing, she brought material succour. Before she left London she had consulted Dr. Andrew Smith, the head of the Army Medical Board, as to whether it would be useful to take out stores of any kind to Scutari; and Dr. Andrew Smith had told her that "nothing was needed." Even Sidney Herbert had given her similar assurances; possibly, owing to an oversight, there might have been some delay in the delivery of the medical stores, which, he said, had been sent out from England "in profusion," but "four days would have remedied this." She preferred to trust her own instincts, and at Marseilles purchased a large quantity of miscellaneous provisions, which were of the utmost use at Scutari. She came, too, amply provided with money—in all, during her stay in the East, about £7000 reached her from private sources; and, in addition, she was able to avail herself of another valuable means of help. At the same time as herself, Mr. Macdonald, of the *Times*, had arrived at Scutari, charged with the duty of administering the large sums of money collected through the agency of that newspaper in aid of the sick and wounded; and Mr. Macdonald had the sense to see that the best use he could make of the *Times* Fund was to put it at the disposal of Miss Nightingale. "I cannot conceive," wrote an eye-witness, "as I now calmly look back on the first three weeks after the arrival of the wounded from Inkerman, how it could have been possible to have avoided a state of things too disastrous to contemplate, had not Miss Nightingale been there, with the means placed at her disposal by Mr. Macdonald." But the official view was different. What! Was the public service to admit, by accepting outside charity, that it was unable to discharge its own duties without the assistance of private and irregular benevolence? Never I And accordingly when Lord

Stratford de Redcliffe, our ambassador at Constantinople, was asked by Mr. Macdonald to indicate how the *Times* Fund could best be employed, he answered that there was indeed one object to which it might very well be devoted—the building of an English Protestant Church at Pera.

Mr. Macdonald did not waste further time with Lord Stratford, and immediately joined forces with Miss Nightingale. But, with such a frame of mind in the highest quarters, it is easy to imagine the kind of disgust and alarm with which the sudden intrusion of a band of amateurs and females must have filled the minds of the ordinary officer and the ordinary military surgeon. They could not understand it; what had women to do with war? Honest Colonels relieved their spleen by the cracking of heavy jokes about "the Bird"; while poor Dr. Hall, a rough terrier of a man, who had worried his way to the top of his profession, was struck speechless with astonishment, and at last observed that Miss Nightingale's appointment was extremely droll.

Her position was, indeed, an official one, but it was hardly the easier for that. In the hospitals it was her duty to provide the services of herself and her nurses when they were asked for by the doctors, and not until then. At first some of the surgeons would have nothing to say to her, and, though she was welcomed by others, the majority were hostile and suspicious. But gradually she gained ground. Her good will could not be denied, and her capacity could not be disregarded. With consummate tact, with all the gentleness of supreme strength, she managed at last to impose her personality upon the susceptible, overwrought, discouraged, and helpless group of men in authority who surrounded her. She stood firm; she was a rock in the angry ocean; with her alone was safety, comfort, life. And so it was that hope dawned at Scutari. The reign of chaos and old night began to dwindle; order came upon the scene, and common sense, and forethought, and decision, radiating out from the little room off the great gallery in the Barrack Hospital where, day and night, the Lady Superintendent was at her task. Progress might be slow, but it was sure. The first sign of a great change came with the appearance of some of those necessary objects with which the hospitals had been unprovided for months. The sick men began to enjoy the use of towels and soap, knives and forks, combs and tooth-brushes. Dr. Hall might snort when he heard of it, asking, with a growl, what a soldier wanted with a tooth-brush; but the good work went on. Eventually the whole business of purveying to the hospitals was, in effect, carried out by Miss Nightingale. She alone, it seemed, whatever the contingency, knew where to lay her hands on what was wanted; she alone could dispense her stores with readiness; above all she alone possessed the art of circumventing the pernicious influences of official etiquette. This was her greatest enemy, and sometimes even she was baffled by it. On one occasion 27,000 shirts, sent out at her instance by the Home Government, arrived, were landed, and were only waiting to be unpacked. But the official "Purveyor" intervened; "he could not unpack them," he said, "without a Board." Miss Nightingale pleaded in vain; the sick and wounded lay half-naked shivering for want of clothing; and three weeks elapsed before the Board released the shirts. A little later, however, on a similar occasion, Miss Nightingale felt that she could assert her own authority. She ordered a Government consignment to be forcibly opened, while the miserable "Purveyor" stood by, wringing his hands in departmental agony.

Vast quantities of valuable stores sent from England lay, she found, engulfed in the bottomless abyss of the Turkish Customs House. Other ship-loads, buried beneath munitions of war destined for Balaclava, passed Scutari without a sign, and thus hospital materials were sometimes carried to and fro three times over the Black Sea, before they reached their destination. The whole system was clearly at fault, and Miss Nightingale suggested to the home authorities that a Government Store House should be instituted at Scutari for the reception and distribution of the consignments. Six months after her arrival this was done.

In the meantime she had reorganised the kitchens and the laundries in the hospitals. The ill-cooked hunks of meat, vilely served at irregular intervals, which had hitherto been the only diet for the sick men were replaced by punctual meals, well-prepared and appetising, while strengthening extra foods—soups and wines and jellies ("preposterous luxuries," snarled Dr. Hall)—were distributed to those who needed them. One thing, however, she could not effect. The separation of the bones from the meat was no part of official cookery: the rule was that the food must be divided into equal portions, and if some of the portions were all bone—well, every man must take his chance. The rule, perhaps, was not a very good one; but there it was. "It would require a new Regulation of the Service," she was told, "to bone the meat." As for the washing arrangements, they were revolutionised. Up to the time of Miss Nightingale's arrival the number of shirts which the authorities had succeeded in washing was seven. The hospital bedding, she found, was "washed" in cold water. She took a Turkish house, had boilers installed, and employed soldiers' wives to do the laundry work. The expenses were defrayed from her own funds and that of the Times; and henceforward the sick and wounded had the comfort of clean linen.

Then she turned her attention to their clothing. Owing to military exigencies the greater number of the men had abandoned their kit; their knapsacks were lost for ever; they possessed nothing but what was on their persons, and that was usually only fit for speedy destruction. The "Purveyor," of course, pointed out that, according to the regulations, all soldiers should bring with them into hospital an adequate supply of clothing, and he declared that it was no business of his to make good their deficiencies. Apparently, it was the business of Miss Nightingale. She procured socks, boots, and shirts in enormous quantities; she had trousers made, she rigged up dressing-gowns. "The fact is," she told Sidney Herbert, "I am now clothing the British Army."

All at once, word came from the Crimea that a great new contingent of sick and wounded might shortly be expected. Where were they to go? Every available inch in the wards was occupied; the affair was serious and pressing, and the authorities stood aghast. There were some dilapidated rooms in the Barrack Hospital, unfit for human habitation, but Miss Nightingale believed that if measures were promptly taken they might be made capable of accommodating several hundred beds. One of the doctors agreed with her; the rest of the officials were irresolute: it would be a very expensive job, they said; it would involve building; and who could take the responsibility? The proper course was that a representation should be made to the Director-General of the Army Medical Department in London; then the Director-General would apply to the Horse Guards, the Horse Guards would move the Ordnance, the Ordnance would lay the matter before the Treasury, and, if the Treasury gave its consent, the work might be correctly carried through, several months after the necessity for it had disappeared. Miss Nightingale, however, had made up her mind, and she persuaded Lord Stratford—or thought she had persuaded him—to give his sanction to the required expenditure. A hundred and twenty-five workmen were immediately engaged, and the work was begun. The workmen struck; whereupon Lord Stratford washed his hands of the whole business. Miss Nightingale engaged two hundred other workmen on her own authority, and paid the bill out of her own resources. The wards were ready by the required date; five hundred sick men were received in them; and all the utensils, including knives, forks, spoons, cans and towels, were supplied by Miss Nightingale.

This remarkable woman was in truth performing the function of an administrative chief. How had this come about? Was she not in reality merely a nurse? Was it not her duty simply to tend to the sick? And indeed, was it not as a ministering angel, a gentle "lady with a lamp" that she actually impressed the minds of her contemporaries? No doubt that was so; and yet it is no less certain that, as she herself said, the specific business of nursing was "the least important of the functions into which she had been forced." It was clear that in the state of disorganisation into which the hospitals at Scutari had fallen the most pressing, the really vital, need was for something more than nursing; it was for the necessary elements of civilised life—the commonest material objects, the most ordinary cleanliness, the rudimentary habits of order and authority. "Oh, dear Miss Nightingale," said one of her party as they were approaching Constantinople, "when we land, let there be no delays, let us get straight to nursing the poor fellows!" "The strongest will be wanted at the wash-tub," was Miss Nightingale's answer. And it was upon the wash-tub, and all that the wash-tub stood for, that she expended her greatest energies. Yet to say that is perhaps to say too much. For to those who watched her at work among the sick, moving day and night from bed to bed, with that unflinching courage, with that indefatigable vigilance, it seemed as if the concentrated force of an undivided and unparalleled devotion could hardly suffice for that portion of her task alone. Wherever, in those vast wards, suffering was at its worst and the need for help was greatest, there, as if by magic, was Miss Nightingale. Her superhuman equanimity would, at the moment of some ghastly operation, nerve the victim to endure and almost to hope. Her sympathy would assuage the pangs of dying and bring back to those still living something of the forgotten charm of life. Over and over again her untiring efforts rescued those whom the surgeons had abandoned as beyond the possibility of cure. Her mere presence brought with it a strange influence. A passionate idolatry spread among the men: they kissed her shadow as it passed. They did more. "Before she came," said a soldier, "there was cussin' and swearin', but after that it was as 'oly as a church." The most cherished privilege of the fighting man was abandoned for the sake of Miss Nightingale. In those "lowest sinks of human misery," as she herself put it, she never heard the use of one expression "which could distress a gentlewoman."

She was heroic; and these were the humble tributes paid by those of grosser mould to that high quality. Certainly, she was heroic. Yet her heroism was not of that simple sort so dear to the readers of novels and the compilers of hagiologies—the romantic sentimental heroism with which mankind loves to invest its chosen darlings: it was made of sterner stuff. To the wounded soldier on his couch of agony she might well appear in the guise of a gracious angel of mercy; but the military surgeons, and the orderlies, and her own nurses, and the "Purveyor," and Dr. Hall, and even Lord Stratford himself could tell a different story. It was not by gentle sweetness and womanly self-abnegation that she had brought order out of chaos in the Scutari Hospitals, that, from her own resources, she had clothed the British Army, that she had spread her dominion over the serried and reluctant powers of the official world; it was by strict method, by stern discipline, by rigid attention to detail, by ceaseless labour, by the fixed determination of an indomitable will. Beneath her cool and calm demeanour lurked fierce and passionate fires. As she passed through the wards in her plain dress, so quiet, so unassuming, she struck the casual observer simply as the pattern of a perfect lady; but the keener eye perceived something more than that— the serenity of high deliberation in the scope of the capacious brow, the sign of power in the dominating curve of the thin nose, and the traces of a harsh and dangerous temper—something peevish, something mocking, and yet something precise—in the small and delicate mouth. There was humour in the face; but the curious watcher might wonder whether it was humour of a very pleasant kind; might ask himself, even as he heard the laughter and marked the jokes with which she cheered the spirits of her patients, what sort of sardonic merriment this same lady might not give vent to, in the privacy of her chamber. As for her voice, it was true of it, even more than of her countenance, that it "had that in it one must fain call master." Those clear tones were in no need of emphasis: "I never heard her raise her voice," said one of her companions. Only, when she had spoken, it seemed as if nothing could follow but obedience. Once, when she had given some direction, a doctor ventured to remark that the thing could not be done. "But it must be done," said Miss Nightingale. A chance bystander, who heard the words, never forgot through all his life the irresistible authority of them. And they were spoken quietly—very quietly indeed.

Late at night, when the long miles of beds lay wrapped in darkness. Miss Nightingale would sit at work in her little room, over her correspondence. It was one of the most formidable of all her duties. There were hundreds of letters to be written to the friends and relations of soldiers; there was the enormous mass of official documents to be dealt with; there were her own private letters to be answered; and, most important of all, there was the composition of her long and confidential reports to Sidney Herbert. These were by no means official communications. Her soul, pent up all day in the restraint and reserve of a vast responsibility, now at last poured itself out in these letters with all its natural vehemence, like a swollen torrent through an open sluice. Here, at least, she did not mince matters. Here she painted in her darkest colours the hideous scenes which surrounded her; here she tore away remorselessly the last veils still shrouding the abominable truth. Then she would fill pages with recommendations and suggestions, with criticisms of the minutest details of organisation, with elaborate calculations of contingencies, with exhaustive analyses and statistical statements piled up in breathless eagerness one on the top of the other. And then her pen, in the virulence of its volubility, would rush on to the discussion of individuals, to the denunciation of an incompetent surgeon or the ridicule of a self-sufficient nurse. Her sarcasm searched the ranks of the officials with the deadly and unsparing precision of a machine-gun. Her nicknames were terrible. She respected no one: Lord Stratford, Lord Raglan, Lady Stratford, Dr. Andrew Smith, Dr. Hall, the Commissary-General, the Purveyor—she fulminated against them all. The intolerable futility of mankind obsessed her like a nightmare, and she gnashed her teeth against it. "I do well to be angry," was the burden of her cry. How many just men were there at Scutari? How many who cared at all for the sick, or had done anything for their relief? Were there ten? Were there five? Was there even one? She could not be sure.

At one time, during several weeks, her vituperations descended upon the head of Sidney Herbert himself. He had misinterpreted her wishes, he had traversed her positive instructions, and it was not until he had admitted his error and apologised in abject terms that he was allowed again into favour. While this misunderstanding was at its height an aristocratic young gentleman arrived at Scutari with a recommendation from the Minister. He had come out from England filled with a romantic desire to render homage to the angelic heroine of his dreams. He had, he said, cast aside his life of ease and luxury; he would devote his days and nights to the service of that gentle lady; he would perform the most menial offices, he would "fag" for her, he would be her footman—and feel requited by a single smile. A single smile, indeed, he had, but it was of an unexpected kind. Miss Nightingale at first refused to see him, and then, when she consented, believing that he was an emissary sent by Sidney Herbert to put her in the wrong over their dispute, she took notes of her conversation with him, and insisted on his signing them at the end of it. The young gentleman returned to England by the next ship.

This quarrel with Sidney Herbert was, however, an exceptional incident. Alike by him, and by Lord Panmure, his successor at the War Office, she was firmly supported; and the fact that during the whole of her stay at Scutari she had the Home Government at her back, was her trump card in her dealings with the hospital authorities. Nor was it only the Government that was behind her: public opinion in England early recognised the high importance of her mission, and its enthusiastic appreciation of her work soon reached an extraordinary height. The Queen herself was deeply moved. She made repeated inquiries as to the welfare of Miss Nightingale; she asked to see her accounts of the wounded, and made her the intermediary between the throne and the troops. "Let Mrs. Herbert know," she wrote to the War Minister, "that I wish Miss Nightingale and the 'ladies would tell these poor noble, wounded, and sick men that *no one* takes a warmer interest or feels *more* for their sufferings or admires their courage and heroism *more* than their Queen. Day and night she thinks of her beloved troops. So does the Prince. Beg Mrs. Herbert to communicate these my words to those ladies, as I know that *our* sympathy is much valued by these noble fellows." The letter was read aloud in the wards by the Chaplain. "It is a very feeling letter," said the men.

And so the months passed, and that fell winter which had begun with Inkerman and had dragged itself out through the long agony of the investment of Sebastopol, at last was over. In May, 1855, after six months of labour. Miss Nightingale could look with something like satisfaction at the condition of the Scutari hospitals. Had they done nothing more than survive the terrible strain which had been put upon them, it would have been a matter for congratulation; but they had done much more than that; they had marvellously improved. The confusion and the pressure in the wards had come to an end; order reigned in them, and cleanliness; the supplies were bountiful and prompt; important sanitary works had been carried out. One simple comparison of figures was enough to reveal the extraordinary change: the rate of mortality among the cases treated had fallen from 42 per cent, to 22 per thousand. But still the indefatigable lady was not satisfied. The main problem had been solved—the physical needs of the men had been provided for; their mental and spiritual needs remained. She set up and furnished reading-rooms and recreation-rooms. She started classes and lectures. Officers were amazed to see her treating their men as if they were human beings, and assured her that she would only end by "spoiling the brutes." But that was not Miss Nightingale's opinion, and she was justified. The private soldier began to drink less, and even—though that seemed impossible—to save his pay. Miss Nightingale became a banker for the army, receiving and sending home large sums of money every month. At last, reluctantly, the Government followed suit, and established machinery of its own for the remission of money. Lord Panmure, however, remained sceptical; "it will do no good," he pronounced; "the British soldier is not a remitting animal." But, in fact, during the next six months, £71,000 was sent home.

Amid all these activities, Miss Nightingale took up the further task of inspecting the hospitals in the Crimea itself. The labour was extreme, and the conditions of life were almost intolerable. She spent whole days in the saddle, or was driven over those bleak and rocky heights in a baggage cart. Sometimes she stood for hours in the heavily falling snow, and would only reach her hut at dead of night after walking for miles through perilous ravines. Her powers of resistance seemed incredible, but at last they were exhausted. She was attacked by fever, and for a moment came very near to death. Yet she worked on; if she could not move, she could at least write; and write she did until her mind had left her; and after it had left her, in what seemed the delirious trance of death itself, she still wrote. When, after many weeks, she was strong enough to travel, she was implored to return to England, but she utterly refused. She would not go back, she said, before the last of the soldiers had left Scutari.

This happy moment had almost arrived, when suddenly the smouldering hostilities of the medical authorities burst out into a flame. Dr. Hall's labours had been rewarded by a K.C.B.—letters which, as Miss Nightingale told Sidney Herbert, she could only suppose to mean "Knight of the Crimean Burial-grounds"— and the honour had turned his head. He was Sir John, and he would be thwarted no longer. Disputes had lately arisen between Miss Nightingale and some of the nurses in the Crimean hospitals. The situation had been embittered by rumours of religious dissensions, for, while the Crimean nurses were Roman Catholics, many of those at Scutari were suspected of a regrettable propensity towards the tenets of Dr. Pasey. Miss Nightingale was by no means disturbed by these sectarian differences, but any suggestion that her supreme authority over all the nurses with the Army was in doubt was enough to rouse her to fury; and it appeared that Mrs. Bridgeman, the Reverend Mother in the Crimea, had ventured to call that authority in question. Sir John Hall thought that his opportunity had come, and strongly supported Mrs. Bridgeman—or, as Miss Nightingale preferred to call her, the "Reverend Brickbat." There was a violent struggle; Miss Nightingale's rage was terrible. Dr. Hall, she declared, was doing his best to "root her out of the Crimea." She would bear it no longer; the War Office was playing her false; there was only one thing to be done—Sidney Herbert must move for the production of papers in the House of Commons, so that the public might be able to judge between her and her enemies. Sidney Herbert with great difficulty calmed her down. Orders were immediately despatched putting her supremacy beyond doubt, and the Reverend Brickbat withdrew from the scene. Sir John, however, was more tenacious. A few weeks later, Miss Nightingale and her nurses visited the Crimea for the last time, and the brilliant idea occurred to him that he could crush her by a very simple expedient—he would starve her into submission; and he actually ordered that no rations of any kind should be supplied to her. He had already tried this plan with great effect upon an unfortunate medical man whose presence in the Crimea he had considered an intrusion; but he was now to learn that such tricks were thrown away upon Miss Nightingale. With extraordinary foresight, she had brought with her a great supply of food; she succeeded in obtaining more at her own expense and by her own exertions; and thus for ten days, in that inhospitable country, she was able to feed herself and twenty-four nurses. Eventually the military authorities intervened in her favour, and Sir John had to confess that he was beaten.

It was not until July, 1856—four months after the Declaration of Peace—that Miss Nightingale left Scutari for England. Her reputation was now enormous, and the enthusiasm of the public was unbounded. The royal approbation was expressed by the gift of a brooch, accompanied by a private letter. "You are, I know, well aware," wrote Her Majesty "of the high sense I entertain of the Christian devotion which you have displayed during this great and bloody war, and I need hardly repeat to you how warm my admiration is for your services, which are fully equal to those of my dear and brave soldiers, whose sufferings you have had the *privilege* of alleviating in so merciful a manner. I am, however, anxious of marking my feelings in a manner which I trust will be agreeable to you, and therefore send you with this letter a brooch, the form and emblems of which commemorate your great and blessed work, and which I hope you will wear as a mark of the high approbation of your Sovereign!"

"It will be a very great satisfaction to me," Her Majesty added, "to make the acquaintance of one who has set so bright an example to our sex."

The brooch, which was designed by the Prince Consort, bore a St. George's cross in red enamel, and the Royal cypher surmounted by diamonds. The whole was encircled by the inscription "Blessed are the Merciful."

III

The name of Florence Nightingale lives in the memory of the world by virtue of the lurid and heroic adventure of the Crimea. Had she died—as she nearly did—upon her return to England, her reputation would hardly have been different; her legend would have come down to us almost as we know it to-day—that gentle vision of female virtue which first took shape before the adoring eyes of the sick soldiers at Scutari. Yet, as a matter of fact, she lived for more than half a century after the Crimean War; and during the greater part of that long period all the energy and all the devotion of her extraordinary nature were working at their highest pitch. What she accomplished in those years of unknown labour could, indeed, hardly have been more glorious than her Crimean triumphs; but it was certainly more important. The true history was far stranger even than the myth. In Miss Nightingale's own eyes the adventure of the Crimea was a mere incident—scarcely more than a useful steppingstone in her career. It was the fulcrum with which she hoped to move the world; but it was only the fulcrum. For more than a generation she was to sit in secret, working her lever; and her real life began at the very moment when, in the popular imagination, it had ended.

She arrived in England in a shattered state of health. The hardships and the ceaseless effort of the last two years had undermined her nervous system; her heart was pronounced to be affected; she suffered constantly from fainting-fits and terrible attacks of utter physical prostration. The doctors declared that one thing alone would save her—a complete and prolonged rest. But that was also the one thing with which she would have nothing to do. She had never been in the habit of resting; why should she begin now? Now, when her opportunity had come at last; now, when the iron was hot, and it was time to strike? No; she had work to do; and, come what might, she would do it.

The doctors protested in vain; in vain her family lamented and entreated, in vain her friends pointed out to her the madness of such a course. Madness? Mad—possessed—perhaps she was. A demoniac frenzy had seized upon her. As she lay upon her sofa, gasping, she devoured blue-books, dictated letters, and, in the intervals of her palpitations, cracked her febrile jokes. For months at a stretch she never left her bed. For years she was in daily expectation of Death. But she would not rest. At this rate, the doctors assured her, even if she did not die, she would become an invalid for life. She could not help that; there was the work to be done; and, as for rest, very likely she might rest ... when she had done it.

Wherever she went, in London or in the country, in the hills of Derbyshire, or among the rhododendrons at Embley, she was haunted by a ghost. It was the spectre of Scutari—the hideous vision of the organisation of a military hospital. She would lay that phantom, or she would perish. The whole system of the Army Medical Department, the education of the Medical Officer, the regulations of hospital procedure ... *rest?* How could she rest while these things were as they were, while, if the like necessity were to arise again, the like results would follow? And, even in peace and at home, what was the sanitary condition of the Army? The mortality in the barracks was, she found, nearly double the mortality in civil life. "You might as well take 1100 men every year out upon Salisbury Plain and shoot them," she said. After inspecting the hospitals at Chatham, she smiled grimly. "Yes, this is one more symptom of the system which, in the Crimea, put to death 16,000 men." Scutari had given her knowledge; and it had given her power too: her enormous reputation was at her back—an incalculable force. Other work, other duties, might lie before her; but the most urgent, the most obvious, of all was to look to the health of the Army.

One of her very first steps was to take advantage of the invitation which Queen Victoria had sent her to the Crimea, together with the commemorative brooch. Within a few weeks of her return, she visited Balmoral, and had several interviews both with the Queen and the Prince Consort. "She put before us," wrote the Prince in his diary, "all the defects of our present military hospital system, and the reforms that are needed." She related "the whole story" of her experiences in the East; and, in addition, she managed to have some long and confidential talks with His Royal Highness on metaphysics and religion. The impression which she created was excellent. "Sic gefällt uns sehr," noted the Prince, "ist sehr bescheiden." Her Majesty's comment was different—"Such a *head!* I wish we had her at the War Office."

But Miss Nightingale was not at the War Office, and for a very simple reason: she was a woman. Lord Panmure, however, *was* (though indeed the reason for that was not quite so simple); and it was upon Lord Panmure that the issue of Miss Nightingale's efforts for reform must primarily depend. That burly Scottish nobleman had not, in spite of his most earnest endeavours, had a very easy time of it as Secretary of State for War. He had come into office in the middle of the Sebastopol campaign, and had felt himself very well fitted for the position, since he had acquired in former days an inside knowledge of the Army—as a Captain of Hussars. It was this inside knowledge which had enabled him to inform Miss Nightingale with such authority that "the British soldier is not a remitting animal." And perhaps it was this same consciousness of a command of his subject which had impelled him to write a dispatch to Lord Raglan, blandly informing the Commander-in-Chief in the Field just how he was neglecting his duties, and pointing out to him that if he would only try he really might do a little better next time. Lord Raglan's reply, calculated as it was to make its recipient sink into the earth, did not quite have that effect upon Lord Panmure, who, whatever might have been his faults, had never been accused of being supersensitive. However, he allowed the matter to drop; and a little later Lord Raglan died—worn out, some people said, by work and anxiety. He was succeeded by an excellent red-nosed old gentleman, General Simpson, whom nobody has ever heard of, and who took Sebastopol. But Lord Panmure's relations with him were hardly more satisfactory than his relations with Lord Raglan; for, while Lord Raglan had been too independent, poor General Simpson erred in the opposite direction, perpetually asked advice, suffered from lumbago, doubted, his nose growing daily redder and redder, whether he was fit for his post, and, by alternate mails, sent in and withdrew his resignation. Then, too, both the General and the Minister suffered acutely from that distressingly useful new invention, the electric telegraph. On one occasion General Simpson felt obliged actually to expostulate. "I think, my Lord," he wrote, "that some telegraphic messages reach us that cannot be sent under due authority, and are perhaps unknown to you, although under the protection of your Lordship's name. For instance, I was called up last night, a dragoon having come express with a telegraphic message in these words, 'Lord Panmure to General Simpson—Captain Jarvis has been bitten by a centipede. How is he now?'" General Simpson might have put up with this, though to be sure it did seem "rather too trifling an affair to call for a dragoon to ride a couple of miles in the dark that he may knock up the Commander of the Army out of the very small allowance of sleep permitted him"; but what was really more than he could bear was to find "upon sending in the morning another mounted dragoon to inquire after Captain Jarvis, four miles off, that he never has been bitten at all, but has had a boil, from which he is fast recovering." But Lord Panmure had troubles of his own. His favourite nephew, Captain Dowbiggin, was at the front, and to one of his telegrams to the Commander-in-Chief the Minister had taken occasion to append the following carefully qualified sentence—"I recommend Dowbiggin to your notice, should you have a vacancy, and if he is fit." Unfortunately, in those early days, it was left to the discretion of the telegraphist to compress the messages which passed through his hands; so that the result was that Lord Panmure's delicate appeal reached its destination in the laconic form of "Look after Dowb." The Headquarters Staff were at first extremely puzzled; they were at last extremely amused. The story spread; and "Look after Dowb" remained for many years the familiar formula for describing official hints in favour of deserving nephews.

And now that all this* was over, now that Sebastopol had been, somehow or another, taken, now that peace was, somehow or another, made, now that the troubles of office might surely be expected to be at an end at last—here was Miss Nightingale breaking in upon the scene, with her talk about the state of the hospitals and the necessity for sanitary reform. It was most irksome; and Lord Panmure almost began to wish that he was engaged upon some more congenial occupation—discussing, perhaps, the constitution of the Free Church of Scotland—a question in which he was profoundly interested. But no; duty was paramount; and he set himself, with a sigh of resignation, to the task of doing as little of it as he possibly could.

"The Bison" his friends called him; and the name fitted both his physical demeanour and his habit of mind. That large low head seemed to have been created for butting rather than for anything else. There he stood. four-square and menacing, in the doorway of reform; and it remained to be seen whether the bulky mass, upon whose solid hide even the barbed arrows of Lord Raglan's scorn had made no mark, would prove amenable to the pressure of Miss Nightingale. Nor was he alone in the doorway. There, loomed behind him the whole phalanx of professional conservatism, the stubborn supporters of the out-of-date, the worshippers and the victims of War Office routine. Among these it was only natural that Dr. Andrew Smith, the head of the Army Medical Department, should have been pre-eminent—Dr. Andrew Smith, who had assured Miss Nightingale before she left England that "nothing was wanted at Scutari." Such were her opponents; but she too was not without allies. She had gained the ear of Royalty—which was something; at any moment that she pleased she could gain the ear of the public—which was a great deal. She had a host of admirers and friends; and—to say nothing of her personal qualities—her knowledge, her tenacity, her tact—she possessed, too, one advantage which then, far more even than now, carried an immense weight—she belonged to the highest circle of society. She moved naturally among Peers and Cabinet Ministers—she was one of their own set; and in those days their set was a very narrow one. What kind of attention would such persons have paid to some middle-class woman with whom they were not acquainted, who possessed great experience of army nursing and had decided views upon hospital reform? They would have politely ignored her; but it was impossible to ignore Flo Nightingale. When she spoke, they were obliged to listen; and, when they had once begun to do that—what might not follow? She knew her power, and she used it. She supported her weightiest minutes with familiar witty little notes. The Bison began to look grave. It might be difficult—it might be damned difficult—to put down one's head against the white hand of a lady.

A Chapter from
Eminent Victorians, 1918

A GUIDE TO
HOSPITALS AND NURSING

WRITINGS AND EXCERPTS
BY FLORENCE NIGHTINGALE

SUGGESTIONS ON
A SYSTEM OF NURSING
FOR HOSPITALS IN INDIA.

To the Secretary of the
Sanitary Commission for Bengal.

Sir,

In reply to your letter of November 21, 1864, requesting me to send to you any suggestions which might occur to me regarding the organization of a system of Female Nursing in Indian Hospitals, I beg herewith to transmit a paper of suggestions which I hope may assist you in considering the subject.

In order to supply the requisite number of Nurses for the Hospitals of India, you must have schools for their instruction and training, either in England or in India, or in both. For these schools there must be competent teachers to instruct and train the untaught, and if such teachers cannot at present be found in India, they must be sent from England. Unless it is assumed that the development of excellence in all that relates to nursing will be as rapid and the teaching as good in India as in England, it would be necessary to provide for a continued supply of teachers, that is, of Matrons and Head Nurses, trained at home. No one, probably, who is acquainted with European life in India will doubt that such a continuous stream of fresh blood and advanced knowledge will be necessary to prevent progressive deterioration.

Then, if this be so, you will require a sort of normal school in England at which Matrons and Head Nurses may be thoroughly trained for service in India, not merely as Nurses but as teachers of nursing. A great part of the training must be conducted by the Head Nurses, even where there is a Training Matron. There does not appear to be any other practicable mode of adequately supplying what is required. Whether you train in India or not, the Government of India ought to make arrangements for the training, in England, of Matrons and Head Nurses for service in India, on such a footing as may reasonably be expected to supply annually the number required to keep up, to its full amount, the establishment of Matrons and Head Nurses, trained in Europe, which may be considered desirable.

The inducements which the Government of India would no doubt be prepared to hold out, would probably attract to their service a very competent and trustworthy class of persons, more especially if it were, as it probably ought to be, a "covenanted service" —a service in which employers and employed entered into a formal contract or covenant. In that case what the Government undertook to do would be fixed by regulations which the persons entering the service would engage to observe and the Government would be bound to act up to.

One of the advantages of making it a regular service would be that you might then, to a limited extent, hold out a prospect of promotion, not of course by seniority but by selection for superior merit and distinguished service, in which length of service would be considered. This need not exclude recruiting in India, especially for the ranks. It is probable that in some parts of India persons, either born in this country or of English or Anglo-Indian parentage, and of suitable character and education, might desire to enter such a service, and some of them might rise in it. Such persons might be very useful from their knowledge of the native languages and of local circumstances of which persons arriving from England wrould necessarily be ignorant.

One of the most obvious difficulties, in the way of carrying out any such systematic organization as is above suggested, would arise from the inducements to marry, Which would beset Nurses of all grades in India, and the consequent danger that the Government might thus lose the services of persons who had been trained and conveyed hither at great cost. A certain term of service in India might be made a condition of employment, but if this condition were violated by marriage, dismissal from the service would be no punishment, and would not even involve any sacrifice which the Nurse had not predetermined to make. A breach of the contract might no doubt involve certain penalties, which might be enforced by legal proceedings, but there would probably be a disinclination to prosecute, or, in case of prosecution, to convict or to give adequate damages.

Perhaps the best course might be to annex a specified pecuniary penalty to breach of the contract, by marriage or otherwise, the amount to diminish with each year of service actually performed in India. This might go far to reimburse the Government for the loss of service, and might incline both the Nurse and her suitor to postpone their nuptials until the stipulated term of service should have been completed, for I presume that the husband, on his marriage, would become liable for the amount of the penalty, being a debt due by his wife.

If the attempt to supply the Hospitals of India with female Nurses is not to be a failure, it is plain that it must be made on some organized plan, which, being based on a stable foundation, may be expected to give permanence and efficiency to the system. Were it as easy to find competent Matrons and Head Nurses as it is to find female mill workers, it may be questioned whether it would be advisable to send out a ship load of them at once, to be scattered over the country from Cape Comorin to Peshawur. To place the majority thus beyond the control and guidance of the heads of their own very special department, would be not only to exclude all hope of efficient and uniform organization, but almost to ensure the failure of the majority of them, and with it a discreditable break down of the whole system. But this is a danger that cannot be incurred, for the Nurses do not exist, and years must elapse before a sufficient number can be "made" to supply the Hospitals of India. There is therefore ample time and opportunity to devise a suitable scheme and to pursue it in a tentative manner, correcting and adjusting it as the experiments are being worked out.

At how many stations in India it would be desirable to institute such tentative trials of nursing would depend not only on the local circumstances, but also on the number of competent and suitable persons who could be selected in this country to carry out the scheme. It would be better to begin with one well selected establishment, sufficient only for one Hospital, than to attempt more than one with more doubtful materials. Much no one can foresee how much will depend upon the success of the first attempt. The value of the whole will, in public estimation, be determined by the quality of the first sample that is exhibited. Then the question arises, if there is, at starting, to be only one Hospital nursed, which Hospital ought it to be? There can be no doubt that it ought to be where it will be under the fostering care of the Governor General. Success at Calcutta would probably carry with it public opinion all over India, and would therefore be of greater value than success anywhere else. But assuming that the Government is satisfied that female nursing ought to be provided for the Hospitals of India, and considering that the Government must be the ultimate judges of success or failure, there is no necessity or good reason why that should be desired; and, on the other hand, in carrying out such an experiment it is but just and right, seeing how many difficulties must in any circumstances be encountered, that it should be tried in the circumstances most favourable to success. If it succeeds, the experience acquired there will enable you to extend it, under less favourable circumstances, with a better prospect of success.

In beginning new things we commence with the easier, and having mastered these, proceed to the more difficult.

But this is a question the ultimate decision of which must rest with the Governor General.

On a consideration of the whole circumstances, then, it appears that there are two things which may be set about immediately. First,—to put in operation means of training Matrons and Head Nurses for service in the general Hospitals and the civil and female Hospitals of India, to be employed on such terms and under such conditions as the Government of India may be disposed or induced to offer. Second,—to find a Matron fitted to be the leading pioneer in such a field, and to provide her with a well selected staff of Head Nurses and Nurses capable of showing what nursing really is, to be employed in such Hospital as the Governor General may determine after due consideration. Whatever aid I can give in obtaining suitable Matrons and Nurses shall gladly be given.

The exclusion of all interference with the department of Nurses, so far as relates to discipline, as herein after stated, is obviously indispensable.

The Regulations given may, with trifling modifications, be adopted for India.

If suitable persons can be found, Matrons and Nurses for more than one Hospital might be sent out, and the Governor General would determine to what Hospitals the different Matrons, with their respective establishments, should be sent.

If several matrons, with nursing establishments, are sent out, then a General Superintendent of Nurses should go out at the same time, so that she may hold the reins from the moment of starting. Looking to the extent and population of the Bengal Presidency (including therein the Upper Provinces and the Punjaub), and to the presence of the Governor General, it might be expedient that the three or four Matrons and establishments first formed should be employed there under a General Superintendent for that Presidency. Madras and Bombay could wait for a time.

In case you may consider it advisable to train Nurses in India, I have, in the following suggestions, given such an account of our method of training in England as might enable you to organize a system of training in India.

SUGGESTIONS.

1. The evidence obtained by the Royal Commission on the Sanitary State of the Indian Army and the information contained in the Minute No. 151 of the Sanitary Commission for Bengal show that the systematic introduction of female nursing into Civil, Military General, and Regimental Female Hospitals would be of great service for the sick in India.

2. The evidence shows that the class of women hitherto employed in this work has been of a comparatively humble character, and without due training, while the nursing has been at the same time highly appreciated by the sick.

3. The desirableness of introducing an organized system of nursing is certainly undoubted, and it cannot but excite great satisfaction that the Governor-General in Council has decided that this improvement shall take place.

4. At the beginning of so important a measure, it is to be feared that nothing but difficulties have to be encountered. But there is no reason why these should not be eventually overcome. It is necessary to state this at the commencement, lest any apparent want of success at first should lead to discontinuance of effort.

5. So far as can be seen the difficulties in India will be of the same kind as, but greater in degree, than those we have had to encounter at home. We have had to introduce an entirely new system, to which the older systems of nursing bear but slight resemblance. Our constant feeling has been that the need is universal and that our means are limited, mainly because the study and practice of nursing as a profession, second only in importance to medicine itself, dates only a few years back in England. It exists neither in Scotland nor in Ireland at the present time. And we, out of our limited means, have to supply a trained Nurse or Matron here and there, in the hope that each may become a centre of improvement, however small, until the growing conviction of the importance of the vast field of usefulness which we have opened for women shall supply us

with agents sufficient in number and of such character as will enable us to meet the all but overwhelming demands for help which we receive from all quarters.

6. It will be seen that our means of assisting India directly are at present very limited and yet we are most anxious to send some seed. Good nursing does not grow of itself; it is the result of study, teaching, training, practice, ending in sound tradition which can be transferred elsewhere.

7. The great difficulty to begin with is obtaining suitable material for.training. Even in England, where there is such a constant outcry of want of women's work, comparatively few apply even as candidates for instruction, although we pay all the costs of training, including payments in the name of wages to Probationers. Of those admitted for training, a proportion are found on trial to be unfit. But all our Nurses, to whom we grant certificates, are taken up at once by different Institutions. [We have just sent twelve and a Matron to Liverpool, and are besides training nineteen for Manchester.] And every woman at all competent is at once appointed Matron to a Hospital. It is necessary that at the very beginning the difficulties which have to be met in organizing a system of nursing for India should be known. It is taken for granted that the difficulties in India, to say the very least of it, will not be fewer than ours at home.

8. Supposing, for the sake of argument, that you have the means of training, viz., a capable Matron, Medical Officers willing to help, and suitable material, probably you could not do better than frame your procedure upon a model which has hitherto been found to answer very well, viz., the Rules for admission and training Nurses at St. Thomas's and King's College Hospitals, London, under the "Nightingale Fund." The Probationer Nurses at St. Thomas's are trained in general nursing duties; those at King's College Hospital specially in midwifery and midwifery nursing.

In the process of training, the following are the steps :— A. Every woman applying for admission is required to fill up the

Form of Application, of which is supplied to her by the Matron of St. Thomas's Hospital, on application. B. The Regulations under which the Probationer is admitted to training.

After being received on a month's trial and trained for a month, if the woman shows sufficient aptitude and character, and is herself desirous to complete her training, she is required to come under the subjoined obligation, binding her to enter into Hospital service for at least five years. This is the only recompense the Committee exact for the costs and advantages of training.

The list of "Duties," is put into the hands of every Probationer on entering the service, as a general instruction for her guidance, and she is checked off by the Matron and "Sisters" (Head Nurses) in these same duties.

A Day and Night Time Table, to which all Probationers are required generally to conform.

It prescribes the time of rising, the ward hours, time of meals, time of exercise, hours of rest.

C. From the nature of Midwifery training, it is not practicable to exact the same system at King's College Hospital Midwifery ward as in the regulated wards of St. Thomas's Hospital.

The class of duties required of Midwifery Nurses is also different. These Nurses are chiefly intended for parish work, and are taken up by parochial committees.

They are required, in concert with the parochial or other committee sending them for training, to sign the Agreement, which it will be seen does not restrict them to Hospital practice. It will be seen, from the tenor of the agreement, that committees sending Midwifery Nurses for training pay the cost of maintenance, but all other costs of training are paid out of the "'Fund."

D. The conditions under which Midwifery Probationers are received at King's College Hospital.

E. Once admitted to St. Thomas's Hospital, the Probationer is placed under a Head Nurse (Ward "Sister") having charge of a ward. In addition to her salary received from the Hospital, the

Ward "Sister" is paid by the fund for training these Probationers. The number of Probationers she can adequately train of course depends on the size and arrangement of her ward and its number of beds. The Ward "Sisters" are all under an able Matron, Mrs. Wardroper, who superintends the training of the Probationers, in addition to her other duties, for which the "Fund" pays her 100*l.* a year, irrespective of her salary as Matron to St. Thomas's Hospital. The ward training of the Probationers is thus carried out under the Ward " Sisters" and Matron. To ensure efficiency, each Ward " Sister " is supplied with a Book which corresponds generally with the List of Duties, given to the Probationer on her entrance.

The columns in the Ward " Sister's " Book are filled up by suitable marks once a week.

F. Besides the ward training properly so called, there are a number of duties of a medical and surgical character, in which the Probationers have to be practically instructed. And this instruction is given by the Resident Medical Officer at the bedside or otherwise, for which he is remunerated by the "Fund" at the rate of 50*l.* a year, independently, of course, of his salary as Permanent Medical Officer of the Hospital.

G. St. Thomas's Hospital is the seat of a well-known Medical School, several of the Professors attached to which, voluntarily and without remuneration, give lectures to the Probationers on subjects connected with their special duties, such as elementary instruction in Chemistry, with reference to air, water, food, &c.; Physiology, with reference to a knowledge of the leading functions of the body, and general instruction on medical and surgical topics.

H. At King's College Hospital these instructions are given in midwifery and matters connected with the diseases of women and children, during the time of the special training in midwifery.

I. While the Ward "Sisters " are required to keep a weekly record of the progress of the "Probationers," the Probationers themselves are required to keep a diary of their ward work, in which they write day by day an account of their duties. They are also required to record special cases of disease, injury, or operation, with the daily changes in the case, and the daily alterations in management, such as a Nurse requires to know.

Besides these books, each Nurse keeps notes of the lectures.

All these records kept by the Probationers are carefully examined, and are found to afford important indications of the capabilities of the Probationer.

To show the advantage of this, it has happened that some of the worst educated women have shown a far higher aptitude for nursing than those whose writing and composition evinced their education.

K. A Register is kept by the Matron of St. Thomas's. It will be seen that it corresponds with the Ward Sister's Book and has space for monthly entries during the entire year of training.

L. At the end of the year all the documents are carefully examined by the Committee of the "Nightingale Fund," and the character the Nurse receives is made to correspond as nearly as may be with the results of the training.

We do not give the women a printed certificate, but simply enter the names of all certificated Nurses in the Register as such. This was done to prevent them, in the event of misconduct, from using their certificates improperly. When a Nurse has satisfactorily earned the gratuity attached to her certificate, the Committee, through the Secretary, communicate with her and forward the money.

This system, which has succeeded with us, would apparently, if it were possible to transplant it, work equally well in India. But it is to be feared that this would be difficult at the present time.

The elements required for working such a system of training are:—

a. A good General Hospital.
b. A competent Training Matron (by such a Matron we do not mean a woman whose business is limited to looking

after the linen and housekeeping of the Hospital, either wholly or mostly, but a woman who, whatever may be her duties as Head of the Establishment, performs chiefly and above all others the duty of superintending the nursing of the sick). If in India it is the custom for the Matron to be simply housekeeper, then there must be a separate Training and Nursing Matron (as we are about to establish in one of the largest workhouse infirmaries in the kingdom), and competent to train. The number she could train would depend entirely on the construction of the Hospital, and on the capabilities of the " Head Nurses" or "Ward Sisters" under her.

c. Competent " Head Nurses."

If such are or can be appointed, they should be responsible to the Training Matron; and the Training Matron is not to be responsible in any case to the Housekeeping Matron, [it would, of course, be better that there should be but one Matron, with a Housekeeper subordinate to her.]

The Head Nurses must be competent trainers. Each might perhaps train four Probationers in a properly constructed ward.

Of course the Training Matron, if she is to be herself her only Head Nurse, can only train such a number of Probationers as a Head Nurse could train.

Our period of training is one year for a Nurse, two years for a Head Nurse.

The Training and Nursing Matron should be responsible to the Civil or Military authorities, as the case may be, or to any Committee appointed by them for the purpose.

It has occurred to all that you might find General Hospital accommodation for your principal training establishments at Calcutta, Bombay, and Madras; but in the existing deficiency of materials for training, if all three localities cannot be undertaken, it would be better to confine your attention to Calcutta, to do the work well there, and then to distribute Trained Nurses as Head

Nurses to train others.

10. It is taken for granted that the Medical Officers of Hospitals where training is to be carried on are willing in India, as elsewhere, to render every assistance in their power in aiding the training by oral instruction and bedside work.

11. All Nurses, after training, might be certificated by the Governing Body, in the manner mentioned.

The subjects of training, and the method of record, would apparently be the same in India as here.

12. Sufficient has been said on the subject of training to show that the success of any system must primarily depend upon your obtaining one or more Trained Nurses, themselves capable of training others.

So far as information has been given, you have no one in India at the present time competent for this work.

If it should so happen that we could not send you a good Training Matron, your best way would be to select the most competent woman you have, and act under our method.

But at the best this would be simply a shade better than nothing.

We are so impressed with this, that we have been making inquiries whether we could not help you, even out of our own poverty in agents.

We have been very much pleased to find that the proposal of introducing a Nursing system into India has been received at both our Training Establishments with very great interest, and that every one is ready to help to the very utmost. If volunteers were asked for we believe they could be had; but we have ventured only to raise the question with a view to its being considered by the authorities in India.

13. If you in India should be of opinion that it would be an advantage to have one or two of our Trained Matrons, accompanied by as many Trained Nurses as we can provide, we here will try our best to send them. It would, indeed, be in every way most desirable, if we can accomplish it, to send you a

complete staff, with which you could begin your work of Hospital Nursing as well as of Training at any Hospital you may consider best suited for the object. The usual way of obtaining Nurses trained under the "Nightingale Fund" is to make application to our Training Matron, Mrs. Wardroper, of St. Thomas's Hospital, and Miss Jones, Lady Superintendent of King's College Hospital.

If you see fit to enclose any applications to either of these ladies through me, I will do what is requisite. In order to avoid delay, it would be necessary to state what wages and salaries it is proposed to give, and that the travelling expenses would be paid.

We might not be able to send Nurses at once, because we always require one year at least of completed training, and we are always behindhand with our engagements. In act, the demand is very much beyond our power to supply.

The question has, however, been raised, and we shall be surprised if, before long, suitable women do not volunteer.

We have, as you are aware, a Superintendent-General of Nurses in Military Hospitals, stationed at Netley. One of her duties is training Military Nurses. At present the staff required for home use is incomplete; and none can be spared for India. But it is possible that eventually English Military General Hospitals may be able to supply a certain number of trained Nurses for India. We, however, always consider it necessary that such Nurses should have had training in a Civil as well as in a Military Hospital before they are appointed.

14. The next point of importance is, supposing you supplied with trained Nurses, in what way to organize a Nursing Establishment for the Military Hospitals of India.

a. There must be a Superintendent-General for each Presidency, who must be responsible, directly or indirectly, to the Government of the Presidency.

b. Under this Superintendent-General should be placed all the Nurses of the Presidency, stationed in Hospitals of whatever class, the expenses of which are either partially or wholly paid by Government.

c. The Hospitals into which female Nursing can be most satisfactorily introduced are—

Military General Hospitals.
Civil General Hospitals
Regimental Female Hospitals

d. Wherever there is more than one female Nurse there must be one woman in the position of Matron, and she must, of course, be an European.

e. The European Nurses should be selected and sent off by the SuperintendentGeneral of the Presidency.

f. These European Nurses would require native assistants; and one of their most important duties would be to train these assistants at the Station.

g. It would be most desirable, in the event of any European woman of good character or fair ability presenting herself at any Station, to send her for training to the Training Hospital of the Presidency.

Suppose, then, you have obtained your Superintendent-General, your Hospital Matrons (Superintendents of Nurses), and Nurses, the next important question is the one of government.

In discussing this point, it is necessary to state whom the Nurses should not be under. They should not be under the Medical Officer for discipline. They should be under no male Officer at any Station, i.e. from the time the system is in full operation.

The Superintendent-General of each Presidency should be head of the discipline over all Superintendents and Nurses in all classes of Hospitals; and she herself should be responsible solely to the Government of the Presidency, directly or indirectly.

The Matrons (Superintendents of Nurses) in Hospitals should be directly under the Superintendent-General.

In like manner, the Nurses in each Hospital should be under the Matron (Superintendent) of the Hospital.

i. The duties which each grade has to perform should be laid down by Regulation, and all that the Medical Department or the Governing Body of the Hospital has a right to require is that the Regulation duties shall be faithfully performed.

Any remissness or neglect of duty is a breach of discipline as well as drunkenness or other bad conduct, and can only be dealt with to any good purpose by report to the Matron (Superintendent of Nurses) of the Hospital, and, failing her, to the Superintendent-General of the Presidency.

It is necessary to dwell strongly on this point, because there has been not unfrequently a disposition shown to make the Nursing Establishment responsible on the side of discipline to the Medical Officer, or to the Civil or Military Governor of the Hospital.

Any attempt to introduce such a system in India would be merely to try anew and to fail anew in an attempt which has frequently been made in Europe. In disciplinary matters, a woman only can understand a woman.

It is the duty of the Medical Officer to give what orders, in regard to the sick, he thinks fit to the Nurses. And it is unquestionably the duty of the Nurses to obey or to see his orders carried out.

Simplicity of rules, placing the Nurses in all matters regarding management of sick absolutely under the orders of the Medical men, and in all disciplinary matters absolutely under the female Superintendent, to whom the Medical Officers should report all cases of neglect, is very important. At the outset there must be a clear and recorded definition of the limits of these two classes ofjurisdiction. But neither the Medical Officer nor any other male head should ever have power to punish for disobedience. His duty should end with reporting the case to the female Superior.

k. The duties to be discharged by the Superintendent-General, Superintendents (Matrons), and by Nurses, are fully laid down in the Regulations for General Hospitals, and in the Regulations for Nurses, contained in the new Medical Regulations of the British Army.

These Regulations would apparently answer as they are, or nearly as they are, for Military General Hospitals, in which the heavy duties of the wards would have to be performed in India by male Orderlies or by male native attendants acting under the direction of the Nurse.

In Regimental Female Hospitals, where there would be no male attendants, it would be necessary to place native female attendants at the disposal of the European Nurse, or Matron, to perform certain classes of ward duties.

In Civil Hospitals the male attendants on the male side, and the female attendants on the female side, would have to be placed under the direction of the Trained Nurse or Nurses.

The Regulations would have to be altered to this extent; they would also have to be altered as regards pay, pension, and retirement; and possibly, in some matters of detail, that can only be settled with reference to local customs and experience.

The chief practical point is that, in framing the Regulations for the Nursing Service in Hospitals in India, the British Army Hospital Regulations referred to should be taken as a ground-work, and departed from as little as possible.

l. The great difficulty in the way of government is,—what best to do in the interval between beginning Female Nursing and organizing the Nursing of the Presidency under a Superintendent-General. This will especially be the case as regards Female Regimental Hospitals, where the staff will never be more than two, or at most three, trained Nurses, one of whom must be Matron, but still she will not be of the calibre justly demanded for a Superintendent.

The least of several evils appears to be some such system as that adopted for Female Regimental Hospitals in England, during the transition time until the SuperintendentGeneral can take charge of all Hospitals appertaining to the army. Wherever there is a Female (Military) Hospital in England, a Ladies' Committee is appointed at the station. This Committee takes a general charge of the Hospital and Nursing, and the Medical Officer reports to the Committee any complaints against Matron or Nurses, the Ladies' Committee exercising discipline.

That portion of the War Office Regulations for Female Hospitals at home, bearing on the question of discipline. It is possible that some such organization may answer for securing efficiency among Nurses in Regimental Female Hospitals in India, until a complete system is organized under a Superintendent-General.

We are afraid that the rates of pay in England will hot suffice in India, for various obvious reasons.

To take Military Hospital Nurses, first

Even in England it is found that the pay, beginning at 20/. a year, although it rises by 2/. a year so as to become 30/. per annum after five years' service, is not enough to secure the class of women necessary for this kind of service ; and the Secretary of State for War has been obliged to raise it to 30/. a year for the first year.

These Nurses, of course, receive board, lodging, and an uniform dress, besides pay and pension.

The present Superintendent-General here serves without pay; but this must be always an exceptional case.

As to Superintendents' and Matrons' pay:—

The largest Civil Hospital in London gives 200/. a year and a house.

The others give 150/. and a house, coals, and beer; sometimes a maid, sometimes other privileges.

The Training Matron at St. Thomas's Hospital receives altogether 250/. a year, a house, coals, beer, and other privileges..

Even in England, for any good Training Matron, 200/. a year, quarters, and a maid, is not at all too much.

In our large Civil Hospitals, the Head Nurses receive 50/. or 60/., or even 70/. per annum, with firing, milk, beer, and light, and many other such privileges ; besides one or two rooms, and sometimes a pension.

A good Training Head Nurse is worth her weight in gold. She cannot be easily replaced. This rate of pay is not at all too high, even in England.

What it must be in India, where the opportunity of marriage for every decent woman is so much greater, you will be better able to judge.

To meet this contingency, it may be necessary, in obtaining Nurses from England, that some agreement as to service should be entered into, in order that all the trouble and cost of having them out should not be lost by their marrying directly they are out.

A similar risk of loss of service, though not of travelling expenses, would apply to Nurses trained in India.

It is hardly necessary to add that no women but of unblemished character can ever be admitted as Nurses. Hospitals are the worst places to employ penitents in.

In conclusion I would recommend as follows:—

1. If you have a first-rate Nurse of sufficient experience (such a woman as would be accepted as a Matron in a large London Hospital) who could act as Training Matron, place her in a suitable Hospital, obtain for her the best European material for training which may be available on the spot, and let her train as nearly as may be in conformity with the plan described above.

2. If you have no Matron on whom you can rely for training, we here will try to send you one or more, and also as many Trained Nurses as we from time to time may be able to spare, on receiving application in the manner already mentioned, stating salary, &c.

If you receive a Nursing Staff with its Matron from England, it will be better to place it complete at the Hospital you may select, so that you may have an example of efficient nursing, as well as a Training School for Nurses.

3. The best manner of extending the system of nursing with Nurses trained in India will be to place a Matron and two Nurses at least at each of the larger Hospitals, there to nurse the sick and to train other Nurses, European or native. But the more complete you can make the Nursing Staff for any new Hospital

at the beginning, the greater will be your chance of success.

4. Whatever interim method of government you may find it necessary to adopt for your nursing establishment, you should, as soon as circumstances admit, organize a system of nursing for each Presidency under a Superintendent-General, a Matron (Superintendent of Nurses) for each Hospital, and Hospital Nurses.

5. The Regulations under which the various duties of these Officers are to be performed, should be based on and approximate as nearly as possible to the Regulations for Nurses in Her Majesty's Hospitals, already mentioned.

FLORENCE NIGHTINGALE.

London,
February 24, 1865.

TRAINED NURSING
FOR THE SICK POOR

―――――――――――――

A Letter Addressed to
The Times of Good Friday, April 14, 1876.

The beginning has been made, the first crusade has been fought and won, to bring—a truly 'national' undertaking—real nursing, trained nursing—to the bedsides of cases wanting real nursing among the London sick poor, in the only way in which real nurses can be so brought to the sick poor; and this is by providing a real home, within reach of their work, for the nurses to live in—a home which gives what real family homes are supposed to give—materially, a bedroom for each, dining and sitting-rooms in common, all meals prepared and eaten in the home; morally, direction, support, sympathy in a common work; further training and instruction in it; proper rest and recreation; and a head of the home, who is also and pre-eminently trained and skilled head of the nursing: in short, a home where any good mother, of whatever class, would be willing to let her daughter, however attractive or highly educated, live.

But all this costs money.

WHAT A DISTRICT NURSE IS TO BE.

Allow an old nurse to say her word on this system, which twenty years ago was a paradox, twenty years hence will be a commonplace.

If a nurse has to 'find herself,' to cook for herself, when she comes home 'dog tired' from her patients, to do everything for herself, she cannot do real nursing; for nursing requires the most undivided attention of anything I know, and all the health and strength both of mind and body.

If, then, she has to provide for herself, she can only be half a nurse, and one of two things happens. Either she *is* of the level of her patients, or she sinks to the level of her patients, and actually makes apologies for their dirt and disorderliness, instead of remedying these, and instead of their making apologies to her, and being anxious for these to be remedied. Nay, as the old hospital nurse did thirty years ago, she may even come to prey upon what is provided for her patients.

There is a third alternative: that she breaks her heart.

But *the* thing which always does happen is, that no woman really fit for the work will do it, or ought to do it.

To have a person fit to live in a home—and who would have any other?—and to create homes for the poor, for it is nothing less, you must have a home fit for her to live in.

If you give nurses a bad home, or no home at all, you will have only nurses who will live in a bad home, or no home at all.

They forget what a home is.

How, then, can they reform and recreate, as it were, the homes of the sick poor?

The very thing that we find in these poor sick is, that they lose the feeling of what it is to be clean. The district nurse has to show them their room clean for once; in other words, to do it herself, to sweep and dust away, to empty and wash out all the appalling dirt and foulness; to air and disinfect, rub the windows, sweep the fireplace, carry out and shake the bits of old sacking and carpet, and lay them down again, fetch fresh water and fill the kettle; wash the patient and the children, and make the bed.

Every home she has thus cleaned has always been kept so. This is her glory. She found it a pig-sty; she left it a tidy, airy room.

In fact these nurses are so far above their patients, that the poor are 'ashamed that we should see their homes dirty again.'

One woman burst into tears as she said:

'It looks like it did before I was taken ill, and all my troubles came upon me; indeed I used to be clean and tidy, ask the neighbours if I wasn't; but what with sickness and trouble, I let one thing after another get behind, and then it was too much for me altogether. Why, I haven't been able to make my bed properly since I came out of hospital, for I did not seem to have heart or strength to do anything, but I will *never* let it get into such a state again.'

And she kept her word, the nurse helping daily in the heavier part of the work, when attending to dress the patient's wound, till the woman was able to do it all herself.

In another case, the mother had been two years in bed. The place was a den of foulness. One could cut the air with a knife. The nurse employed two of the little children to collect the foul litter and dirty linen from under the bed and sort it, emptied utensils which had not been emptied for a fortnight (this is common), cleaned the grate, and carried away the caked ashes, washed the children, combed and cleansed their hair, crowded with vermin. Next day, the eldest girl of eight had scoured the place and, perched on a three-legged stool, was trying to wash the dirty linen with her poor little thin arms. A woman, a neighbour, was found to do this.

But the highest compliment of all has to be told. In another den of dirt, Miss Lees, the 'head nurse' was proceeding, after the other most necessary operations, to wash a little puny boy, when he exclaimed: '*Willie don't like to be bathed. Oo may bath de Debil if oo like.*' Such was Willie's opinion of the extraordinary powers of this new nurse: she could wash black white.

How has the tone and state of hospital nurses been raised?

By, more than anything else, making the hospital such a home as good young women—educated young women—can live and nurse in; and, secondly, by raising hospital nursing into such a profession as these can earn an honourable livelihood in.

If this is the case for hospitals, how much more so for district nursing, where the nurses have to be out in all weathers, and not in cab or 'bus, and where must be created, for there is not now, the *esprit de corps* which inspires the nurses of a good hospital and training-school as it does the soldiers of a regiment of many battles and well-worn colours whose glory has to be kept untarnished.

Even now, except in some remarkable instances, the hospital nurse wants more and gets less of the helps, moral, material, and spiritual, than the woman in a good home or service.

The district nurse wants yet more than the hospital nurse, for her life is harder and more exposed: and gets none.

Woman cannot stand alone (though for that matter, still less can men).

Everybody knows how easy it is to sink to the lowest—'it is all the way down hill,' as I heard an old man say—how hard to rise to the highest!

A first beginning has been made to the district London nurse the real help and the real home which are the secret of the success of active religious sisterhoods abroad—together with he real independence, enterprise, indomitable pluck, self reliance, capability of training all the powers to the best efficiency, which are the secret of the success of the highest British character, and all of which are wanted in the crusade against dirt and fever nests—the crusade to let light and air and cleanliness into the worst rooms of the worst places of sick London.

To set these poor sick people going again, with a sound and clean house, as well as with a sound body and mind, is about as great benefit as can be given them—worth acres of gifts and relief.

This *is* depauperising them.

But to train and provide such District Nurses and such District Homes costs money.

WHAT A DISTRICT NURSE IS TO DO.

A nurse is, first, to nurse.

Secondly, to nurse the room as well as the patient—to put the room into nursing order. That is, to make the room such as a patient *can* recover in; to bring care and cleanliness into it, and to teach the inmates to keep up that care and cleanliness.

Thirdly, to bring such sanitary defects as produce sickness and death, and which can only be remedied by the public officer, to the notice of the public whom it concerns.

A nurse cannot be a cook (though 'sweet Jack Falstaff' says she is), a relieving-officer, district-visitor, letter-writer, general storekeeper, upholsterer, almoner, purveyor, Lady Bountiful, head dispenser, and medical comforts shop. A District Nurse can rather less than a hospital nurse be all this. Though, where things are wanting and wanted for recovery, she or her Head knew how and where to apply for them. There are agencies for all these things.

'Upon the written order of the parish doctor, we generally obtain from the workhouse authorities, for those patients whose state requires such nourishment, a supply of meat, brandy, wine, &c., and when we have found a difficulty in obtaining these from the parish authorities, the clergy, district visitors, and charitable missions have supplied us with them, as well as with linen and other necessaries. In some cases the nurses have prepared such nourishment as beef-tea, light puddings, and cooling drinks at the homes of the patients; in others they have been prepared in the Central Home; but usually medical comforts of this kind have been made (as well as given) by the district visitors. In no case has any nurse *given* anything to the patient beyond the actual nursing rendered them; but if as a nurse I am capable of judging nurses' work, I feel I may fairly say that this service has been of a higher character than that rendered by any other nurses in the kingdom,'—*Extract from First Quarterly Report of Miss Florence Lees, Superintendent-General.*

One may pretty safely say that, if district nurses begin by giving relief, they will end by doing nothing but giving relief.

Now, it is utter waste to have a highly trained and skilled nurse to do this; without counting the demoralising and pauperising influence on the sick poor, who have too many such influences already.

How often a drinking man will go *all to drink*, if you support as well as nurse his sick wife, is perhaps little thought of—as also what efforts such a man will make *not* to drink, when his wife is sick, if you help himself and her; to maintain his independence—and if you make his home by cleanliness and care less intolerable.

Perhaps sickness is sent for this very end; and you frustrate it.

The present Association wants to foster the spirit of work (not relief) in the district nurse, and for her to foster the same in her sick poor.

Nor are these District Nurses without hearing and receiving evidence that this spirit is now becoming really understood among their sick.

One poor old woman was heard saying to her younger neighbour: 'Them nurses is real blessings; now husbands and fathers did ought to pay a penny a week, as ud' give us a right to call upon they nurses when we wants they.'

This is the real spirit of the thing.

So nothing is *given* but the nursing, and some day, let us hope that the old woman's sensible plan will be carried out. In the meantime, nurses are nurses—not cooks, nor yet almoners, nor relieving officers. But if needed, they are procured from the proper agencies, and sick comforts made as well as given by these agencies.

(1) A District Nurse must first nurse. She must be of a yet higher class and of a yet fuller training than a hospital nurse because she has not the docter always at hand; because she has no hospital appliances at hand at all; and because she has to take notes of the case for the doctor, who has no one but her to report to him. She is his staff of clinical clerks, dressers, and nurses.

These District Nurses—and it is the first time it has ever been done—keep records of the patient's state, including pulse, temperature, &c., for the doctor. One doctor stated that he knew when an operation ought to be performed by reading the nurse's report on the case; another, that by hearing the nurse's history of the case, he found patients to be suffering from typhoid fever who had been reported as consumptive. And a hospital doctor, who had admitted patients into hospital with the nurses written history of the case, 'doubted if many of our medical students could have sent a better report.'

(2) If a *hospital* must first of all be a place which shall do the sick no harm, how much more must the *sick poor's room* be made a place not to render impossible recovery from the sickness which it has probably bred.

This is what London District Nurses do; they nurse the room as well as the patient, and teach the family to nurse the room.

And it requires a higher stamp of woman to do this; to thus combine the servant with the teacher and with the educated woman who can so command the patient's confidence as to let her do this, than almost any other work.

A well-known bishop, now on the bench, cleaned himself the pig-sties of the Normal Training School, of which he was master, as an example,—perhaps one of the most episcopal acts ever done.

(3) A District Nurse must bring to the notice of the Officer of health, or proper authority, sanitary defects, which he alone can remedy.

Thus dustbins are emptied, water butts cleaned, water supply and drainage examined and remedied, which looked as if this had not been done for one hundred years.

Hospitals are but an intermediate stage of civilisation. At present hospitals are the only place where the sick poor can be nursed, or, indeed, often the sick rich. But the ultimate object is to nurse all sick at home.

Where can the sick poor in general be sick?

At home: it is there that the bulk of sick cases are.

But where can nurses be trained for them?

In hospitals: it is there only that skilled nurses can be trained.

All this makes real nursing of the sick at home the most expensive kind of nursing at present.

Yet no one would wish to convey the whole sick population into hospital, even were it possible, and even if it did not often break up the poor man's home.

In one case Miss Lees' trained nursing enabled the parish doctor to perform a very serious operation in the woman's own home, whereby the parish was saved a guinea a week, and the poor woman's home was saved from being broken up.

But all this costs money. The District Nurses cost money, and the District Home costs money. Each district nurse must have, before she is qualified:—

1. A month's trial in district work.
2. A year's training in hospital nursing.
3. Three months' training in district nursing,
   under the Superintendent-General.

Each District Home must have a superintendent, who initiates and supervises the nurses' work. Moreover, only a limited number of nurses can be placed in one District Home, for more would be too far from their work. The multiplication of homes will cost money.

For anything like a 'National,' or even a 'Metropolitan' concern, a capital of £20,000 and an income of £5,000 a year are wanted.

Of this a great part is wanted at once—

To set on foot three District Homes;

To pay and maintain their superintendents,
   nurses and probationers;

To create a hospital training-school in which to train.

What has been done at present to establish one District Home (which it is hoped will be the Central Home of many other districts) under the charge and training of Miss Florence Lees, as Superintendent-General, with five hospital-trained nurses and three nurse candidates, and to carry on the previously existing work of the East London Nursing Society with six nurses.

The Central Home was opened at 23, Bloomsbury Square in December last, the nursing work having been begun in the neighbourhood, from a temporary abode, in July. The Nightingale Training School at St. Thomas's Hospital is at present giving the year's hospital training to six, to be increased to twelve, admitted candidates.

A group of districts is now about to be nursed where the residents have engaged to raise £300 a year towards the expenses of a district home, with a skilled superintendent for supervising the nursing of four or more trained nurses, and one or two servants; for district nurses have quite other things to do than to cook for and wait upon themselves. They are the servants, and very hard-worked servants, of the poor sick.

We ask the public not to add one more charity or relief agency to the many there are already, but to support a charity—truly 'metropolitan' in its scope, and truly 'national' if carried out—which never has been before.

FLORENCE NIGHTINGALE

April 1876.

WORKHOUSE NURSING

THE STORY OF A SUCCESSFUL EXPERIMENT.

By Florence Nightingale, 1867

The following pages contain a brief account of the experiment successfully tried by the Select Vestry of Liverpool (the guardians of the poor)—the introduction of trained Nurses into the male wards of the Workhouse Infirmary. That experiment having resulted so successfully as to induce the Vestry to extend the system to the remainder of the infirmary, it may be interesting to those who are concerned in the management of workhouses elsewhere to learn something of its history and progress. It is the writer's object to explain—

1. The grounds on which the Vestry were led to undertake the experiment, as stated in the preliminary report of Mr. Carr, the governor, and that of the sub-committee of the Vestry appointed to consider the proposed scheme; and the replies received to inquiries addressed by them to institutions and persons connected with the training and employment of skilled nurses in London and Liverpool, with letters on the subject from Miss Nightingale and Sir John McNeill.

2. The results of the experiment, so far as hitherto ascertained.

The Liverpool Vestry had previously made considerable efforts to improve the workhouse infirmaries. The medical men had been encouraged to make requisition for every material appliance that could facilitate the cure of the sick; and paid female officers were appointed at the rate of one to each 150 or 200 beds, to superintend the giving of medicines and stimulants, and so forth: but of course so small a number, even had they been trained nurses, could do no real nursing, and could exercise little supervision over the twenty drunken or unreliable pauper nurses who were under the nominal direction of each paid officer. An appeal was made to the Vestry to consummate the good work they had thus partially commenced, and it was urged that Liverpool should assume the lead in the task of workhouse reform. The following considerations were submitted to the Select Vestry:—

"That Liverpool could commence this movement with great effect, and with the certainty that her example would be widely followed.

"That she had in times past taken a leading part in such reform. The introduction of the New Poor Law produced little change in Liverpool; so many of its wisest provisions were already in operation there, some of them for twenty or thirty years.

"That she had already established a system of attention to the sick poor in their own houses, which, if only by restoring heads of families to health and work, saved the parish many times the sum that it cost to private benevolence.

"That, lastly and especially, the proposed reform ought to commence in Liverpool, because in her workhouse the guardians had already, by their liberality, provided the sick with everything in the shape of diet and medical comforts that could conduce to recovery; and what was now wanting to give effect to their wise benevolence was, that their system should be administered and their intentions carried out by efficient and reliable nurses, in the stead of unreliable paupers."

The appeal further urged that—

"Successful efforts have been made in many directions to improve the nursing of the sick, and the workhouses must soon be the object of similar endeavours. Those poor sufferers whose disease is protracted and hopeless are refused admission into ordinary hospitals, and must come to the workhouse; and the mere duration of the illness is in such cases sufficient to reduce to poverty the most industrious, careful, and temperate—men who, while they could work, paid regularly their contribution to the poor-rate. Surely, these are entitled to at least as great care as that which sickness at once assures to the imprisoned felon, however criminal, for whom well-paid nurses are provided by the State.

"As to the other class of inmates of the workhouse infirmary—those whose ailments are curable—mere economy requires that the most efficient means should be taken to cure them as speedily as possible, so as to preserve them and their families from becoming paupers.

"Thus justice and expediency alike counsel the introduction into the workhouse of the best known system of nursing. Probably nothing which the skill and kindness of medical men can do, no food or physical appliances which the guardians can supply, no oversight or care which they, acting through pauper nurses, can bring to bear, are wanting in the Liverpool workhouse; but it is to be feared that much of this care, liberality, and thought fails of its object for want of a sufficient number of reliable and duly qualified nurses to carry out the instructions given, to administer food and medicine to the patients, to dress their wounds, and so forth."

This appeal was supported by two letters of Miss Nightingale and Sir John McNeill, G.C.B., President of the Board of Supervision (the Scotch Poor Law Board).

Letter from Miss Nightingale.

115, Park Street, W.
February 5, 1864.

My dear Sir,

I will not delay another day expressing how much I admire, and how deeply I sympathize with the Workhouse plan.

First let me say that Workhouse sick and Workhouse Infirmaries require quite as much care as (I had almost said more than) Hospital sick. There is an even greater work to be accomplished in Workhouse Infirmaries than in Hospitals.

In days long ago, when I visited in one of the largest London Workhouse Infirmaries, I became fully convinced of this.

How gladly would I have become the Matron of a Workhouse.

But of a Visitor's visit, the only result is to break the Visitor's heart. She sees how much could be done and cannot do it.

Liverpool is of all places the one to try this great Reform in. Its example is sure to be followed. It has an admirable body of Guardians; it is a thorough practical people; it has, or soon will have again, money. Lord Russell once said (what is quite true), that the Poor Law was never meant to supersede private charity.

But whatever may be the difficulties about Pauperism, in two things most people agree—viz. that Workhouse sick ought to have the best practical nursing, as well as Hospital sick—and that a good wise Matron may save many of these from life-long pauperism, by first nursing them well, and then rousing them to exertion, and helping them to employment.

In such a scheme as is wisely proposed, there would be four elements.

1. The Guardians, one of whose functions is to
   check pauperism. They could not be expected

    to incur greater cost than at present, *unless*
    it is proved that it cures or saves life.
2. The Visiting or Managing Committee of the
    Guardians, whose authority must not (and
    need not) in any way be interfered with.
3. The Governor, the Medical Officer, and Chaplain.
4. (And under the Governor) the proposed
    Superintendent of Nurses and her nursing staff.
There is no reason why all these parts of the
    machine should not work together.
The funds are provided to pay the extra nursing for a time.
The difficulty is to find the Lady to govern it.

When appointed, she must be authorized— indeed appointed— by the Guardians. She must be their Officer; and must be invested by the Governor with authority to superintend her Nurses in conformity with regulations to be agreed upon.

So far, I see no more difficulty than there was in settling our relations as Nurses to the government officials in the Crimean War.

The cases are somewhat similar.

As to the funds, it is just possible that eventually the Guardians might take all the cost on themselves, as soon as they saw the great advantages and economy of good nursing.

If Liverpool succeeds, the system is quite sure to extend itself.

The Fever Hospital is one of the Workhouse Infirmaries. That is the place to shew what skilful nursing can do. The patients are not all paupers. How many families might be rescued from pauperism by saving the lives of their heads, and by helping the hard-working to more speedy convalescence!

Hopefully yours,

(*Signed*)
FLORENCE NIGHTINGALE.

Extract from a letter from the
Right Honourable Sir John McNeill, G.C.B.,
dated Granton House, Edinburgh, 28th Feb., 1864.

There can be no doubt, I think, that it would be a mistake to have pauper nurses mixed up with paid nurses, and I think I expressed that opinion when we conversed about those things. Paupers might, however, be employed to scrub and to do other menial work, under the orders of the paid nurses. If the paid nurses are to do much good they must have a recognised authority in their wards. Without authority there cannot be due responsibility, and things must get into confusion. A nurse carrying out the instructions of the medical officer must have authority to do so, and resistance to that authority must be treated as a breach of discipline.

To put this upon a right footing from the first, would be indispensable to success. The more a nurse does by influence, and kindly influence, the better; but dealing with the promiscuous inmates of a workhouse, the knowledge that there is authority in reserve to be exercised if necessary, prevents the necessity of resorting to it, and makes the patients duly appreciate the kindness which keeps it in reserve.

With regard to all such matters, a great deal will depend upon the good-will, the good sense, and good feeling of the Governor and Matron, but especially of the Governor. He can do much to promote or to mar the success of the experiment, and so can the medical men; but if they be men of sense and right feeling, they cannot fail to perceive how vast an addition to their own comfort the permanent establishment of such a system as you propose to introduce experimentally, must produce.

The position of a medical man dependent for the execution of his instructions upon nurses who are neither intelligent nor trustworthy, is very painful, and tends to deteriorate his own character, both as a man and as a practitioner, by rendering him callous to preventible suffering which he is denied the proper means of relieving, and by compelling him to forego the use of remedies which require intelligence and conscientious care in administering them. The house Governor, if he be a conscientious man, must be kept in continual anxiety about the conduct of ignorant, and often worthless pauper nurses in the hospital, and is driven at length to be satisfied with a low moral and intellectual standard in the nurses, and a corresponding standard of care and comfort in the hospital.

The Select Vestry took the subject into their serious consideration, and instituted most careful inquiries in various quarters. Among other steps, they called for a report on the probable operation of the proposed system from Mr. Carr, the Governor of the Workhouse. That report ran as follows:—

Extract from the Journal
of the Governor of the Workhouse.

Liverpool,
Thursday, April 14, 1864.

In compliance with the instructions of the Workhouse Committee, I have carefully considered the proposal made to the Committee by a Liverpool gentleman, on the subject of nursing the sick in the Workhouse Hospital, and beg in reference thereto to report—

That, practically, the proposal amounts to this—that there shall not be any pauper nurses in the hospital, but that there shall be appointed in lieu a staff of duly qualified paid nurses and servants, with a head superintendent, under whom the whole of the nursing of the sick shall be conducted on the best known principles.

This proposal rests its claim to favourable consideration on the presumption that the present system of nursing the sick in the Workhouse Hospital is defective. The Committee are aware what that system is. It may thus be briefly stated. Certain wards of the workhouse are set apart as hospital wards. They do not form an hospital worked as a whole, but are divided into five portions, each forming a distinct set of wards, in close proximity to the wards of the healthy paupers, and in five different parts of the workhouse. These five sets of wards I shall call the Workhouse Hospital. The hospital is divided into eleven sections. At the head of each section there is an intelligent paid superintendent nurse, and under each such superintendent nurse there is placed a staff of pauper nurses, with the aid of whom she is required to work her division, according to certain rules and regulations made and provided for that purpose. A copy of these rules is appended hereto; from which it will be seen that the burden of the responsibility of carrying out the orders of the medical officers, devolves upon the head nurses or superintendents of divisions. The pauper nurses clean up the wards, carry the food, and give general assistance to the superintendent—the duties of nursing in detail, that is to say, the bedside nursing, falling chiefly upon them. They are not permitted, however, to serve any patient with stimulants, beer, porter, or medicines requiring exactness or care; all such duties are discharged by the superintendent nurse. The proposal now made to the Committee, means that the paid staff shall be increased, so that the sick shall be cared for by responsible officers only, and not left, even partially, to the care of pauper nurses.

There is no doubt that pauper nurses are unreliable, inefficient, and many of them very worthless; and it is only by careful watching, and the utmost stringency of regulations, that they can be made serviceable in the hospital. No stringency of regulations, however, could guard against the most flagrant abuses, if these women were employed to discharge duties of trust, such as serving out the stimulants, &c. so that their services in attending upon the sick are limited and common-place. There is therefore, in my mind, no doubt, and I cannot see how any doubt can exist, that to remove these women, and appoint in their places women of character, trained as nurses, will tend to improve the position of the sick, and more rapidly restore many of them to health.

To displace these pauper women, however, involves a complete change in all the hospital arrangements, and suggests the difficulty of finding and keeping up a supply of suitable nurses to undertake the work at, as it would no doubt often happen, short notice. The Committee are aware, too, that owing to the fact that the paupers have hitherto been required to attend upon the sick, the accommodation for paid officers is very limited, and that the adoption of the proposal would render it necessary at once to provide additional rooms for the additional staff. The Committee are also aware that the Workhouse Hospital differs from other hospitals in this—that it forms a part only of a mixed establishment, and that there are great difficulties to be overcome in completely cutting off every connexion or species of intercourse between the hospital departments and the healthy inmates, without which the scheme under consideration could hardly succeed. If any good is to result from the adoption of this proposal, the sick should be placed absolutely and entirely in the hands of a paid staff, without the assistance, in any form, of any one of the pauper inmates. Cut off the hospital department from the healthy wards; and do not, under any pretext, suffer communication between the sick and the healthy, and you strike at the root of every species of workhouse abuse; but if, under any pretext, you suffer a large number of healthy paupers to pass daily into the sick departments, as they now do, the adoption of the proposal will effect little good.

But the question has to be still further investigated on the ground of expense; and it has to be decided the number, pay, allowances, and accommodation of the necessary staff to work it out. Now, although I entertain very strong opinions as to the undesirability of employing paupers to discharge responsible duties of any kind, because to do so destroys the value of the workhouse test, and tends to reconcile them to pauperism; and although I view the particular work of nurse-tending as the very worst kind of work for paupers, inasmuch as, while so employed, they are better fed, have more freedom of action than they otherwise would, and can make their places emolumental— thereby holding out a positive inducement to pauperism; and although I have no doubt that the displacement of these women would be followed by the immediate application for discharges by a large per-centage of them; and although, at this moment, many other weighty considerations press upon me in favour of the immediate adoption of the proposal under consideration, I feel unwilling, in view of the difficulties to be overcome, some of which I have indicated, to incur the weighty responsibility of recommending such a course on my own unaided judgment. I have abstained, therefore, from taking up the question of expense, &c. but take the liberty respectfully to suggest, that a sub-committee be appointed to report upon the whole question in all its details. It shall be my anxious desire and pleasure to assist the labours of such sub-committee by every means in my power.

According to the recommendation of Mr. Carr, a Sub-Committee was appointed, consisting of men of great experience in parochial business, who went up to London, and had interviews with the medical and other officers of the two metropolitan hospitals where nursing has been brought to the greatest perfection—St. Thomas's and King's College Hospitals. Finding that some of these gentlemen wished for more information respecting the Workhouse Hospital system before they would venture to express decided opinions as to the economical results of the proposed reform, the Liverpool Visitors drew up a statement on several points affecting this question, with written inquiries, to which answers were returned, verbally or in writing, by the gentlemen consulted. This statement, with the replies which it elicited, is here given at length:—

STATEMENT AND QUESTIONS OF
THE LIVERPOOL SUB-COMMITTEE.

The population of the Parish of Liverpool is about 270,000.

The expenditure from the poor's-rate in and about the relief of the poor is about 100,000*l*. per annum.

Of this about 40,000*l*. is distributed in out-door relief as money and bread. (Of course sickness is one great cause of persons seeking relief, though to what extent this cause operates, even directly, I cannot on so short a notice ascertain or even estimate.)

The expenses (direct) of treating the out-door sick are:—

Salaries of Medical Officers, &c.	£1,800
Medicines, &c.	1,378
	£3,178

The cost of maintaining the Workhouse Hospital may be estimated as follows:—

Maintenance of Patients	£9,700
Salaries of Medical Officers	485
Medicines, &c	1,050
	£11,235

The Hospital contains accommodation for over 1,000 patients, and has often 1,000 in it. The cases at present are:—

Medical	485
Surgical	345
Fever	120
Smallpox	20

The weekly discharges are from twenty to thirty per cent, of the whole number in the hospital.

The present workhouse staff consists of fourteen paid officers (who are superintendents, but not trained nurses), and about 150 paupers acting as nurses, but not paid. It has been proposed to add a trained hospital matron and trained nurses, such as those trained in the Nightingale School, and assistant nurses, so as to give one trained day-nurse and one paid assistant to about every three pauper nurses, and a trained night-nurse on every flat; it is further proposed to pay the paupers who act as nurses, wages. The cost of this would be about 2,000*l.* per annum.

Does your experience of hospitals lead you to believe that the cost of this improved system would be "in part," "wholly," or "more than" repaid to the ratepayers by curing people more quickly, by curing those who otherwise might have become chronic cases, and by enabling those to resume their work who must otherwise have remained or died, and by thus diminishing the duration or amount of that part of pauperism which is the result of sickness?

REPLIES OF PHYSICIANS, &c.
OF ST. THOMAS'S HOSPITAL.

1. REPLY OF R. H. GOOLDEN, ESQ., M.D.

"I have no doubt but that the plan suggested, if properly carried out, would be in the end a saving to the ratepayers, the restoration to health relieving the parish of constant burdens."

2. REPLY OF JOHN SIMON, ESQ.

"I do not feel myself competent to measure at all exactly what might be the pecuniary result of the proposed system. But in my opinion the substitution of skilled for unskilled attendance would be of great advantage to the sick, and would of course tend to diminish that part of the pauperism which results from sickness."

3. REPLY OF SYDNEY JONES, ESQ., M.D.

"In my opinion the improved system of nursing recommended would amply repay the expense incurred."

4. REPLY OF J. S. BRISTOWE, ESQ., M.D.

"I believe that the introduction of paid nurses into the Liverpool Workhouse Infirmary would be of inestimable benefit to the sick poor received into the institution, and would thus amply justify the expense which it is proposed to incur. I also think it very probable that the cost of nursing would be repaid in many other ways to the ratepayers."

5. REPLY OF EDWARD CLAPTON, ESQ., M.D.

"I believe it would be quite repaid."

REPLIES FROM
THE PHYSICIANS, &C.
OF KING'S COLLEGE HOSPITAL.

1. REPLY OF HENRY SMITH, ESQ,
ASSISTANT SURGEON.

"I believe, from a long experience of hospitals and other institutions, that the cost of an improved system of nursing as proposed for the Liverpool Workhouse Hospital would certainly be 'in part ' repaid by restoring the patients to health more quickly."

2. COPY OF A LETTER FROM MISS JONES, LADY SUPERINTENDENT OF ST, JOHN'S HOUSE NURSING SCHOOLS, AND MATRON OF KINGS COLLEGE HOSPITAL.

King's College Hospital, May 4, 1864.

Dear Sir,

The inclosed paper was sent to me yesterday, with the request that I would obtain from some of the medical staff of this Hospital answers to the question proposed at the end of the paper, in order to enable the Vestry in some degree to judge whether that body would be justified, or otherwise, in sanctioning the introduction to their Workhouse Hospital of an improved system of nursing the sick, at the probable annual money cost named in the inclosed paper. I have accordingly submitted the paper to as many of the medical staff as I could see in the short time.

I inclose a note from Mr. Henry Smith, one of the surgeons, who has had considerable experience as to the loss and gain of good and bad nursing. Dr. Wm. O. Priestly, the Physician Accoucheur to this Hospital, formerly of Middlesex Hospital, had not time during his visit to do more than read the paper and give me a verbal answer. He said, "I have no hesitation in saying that the saving would be certain and great."

The Assistant Physician Accoucheur, who has until last week had charge of the medical patients here, as House Physician (Mr. H. L. Kempthorne), says, "The value of trained efficient nursing cannot be overrated in the management of acute diseases, and especially fevers, and would speak for itself in the saving of life, humanly speaking.

"In chronic cases, the eye of the trained nurse would soon detect the malingerer, and thus save the parish the expense of maintaining one who could well keep himself.

"In the prevention and amelioration of disease this plan would soon show its importance in the effects of cleanliness, ventilation, and other points carried out systematically and intelligently.

"The moral influence of the trained nurses by precept and example must in time diffuse itself through the medium of the pauper nurses to the paupers in hospital, the workhouse, and thence to the parish at large."

I regret my inability to obtain fuller testimony to-day, but professional men are busy, and their visits to the hospital only on stated days.

If I can be of further use in any way, pray command me.

I am, Sir,
Very faithfully yours,

M.J.
Superintendent of St. John's.

After collecting and considering all the information within their reach, the Sub-Committee reported as follows:—

The Sub-Committee appointed on the 14th ultimo to consider and report as to a suggested alteration in the Staff of the Workhouse Hospital, report, That the superiority, as nurses, of trained, experienced, and responsible women to the pauper women upon whom, under the present system, the actual nursing of the sick inmates of the workhouse devolves, is so apparent, that they conceive it to be unnecessary to offer any further observations upon this part of the subject. The points which have mainly occupied your Committee's attention are the following:—

1. The cost of introducing a staff of trained nurses into the Workhouse Hospital, or any portion thereof.
2. The practicability of providing sufficient accommodation in the Workhouse for such an increase of officers.
3. The supply of trained nurses.

1. Your Committee are of opinion that the substitution throughout the Workhouse Hospital of trained nurses, for the present pauper nurses, would involve a direct expenditure of from 2,000*l.* to 2,500*l.* per annum. Should it be decided, in the first instance, to introduce the nurses into the male hospital only, it is probable that a sum of 800*l.* per annum would be found sufficient for the purpose. Evidence has been laid before the Committee to show that in those hospitals where the improved system of nursing has been introduced, the increased cost thereof has been more than compensated for by the saving, from the reduction of the time during which the patients are under treatment—the effect, as is alleged, of good and efficient nursing. Whilst your Committee admit the force of the argument, that if this be so in the case of hospitals, where the sick only are burdens upon the funds of the institution, much more must it be so in the case of the parish, where, as often happens, the whole family are chargeable upon the rates in consequence of the sickness of its head; they think it necessary to point out that one great difference between the workhouse hospital and an ordinary infirmary consists in this, that while in the latter (as a rule) none but acute and supposed curable cases are admitted, the former is, in many cases, the refuge of those who, as incurables, cannot gain admittance to other asylums. There can, however, be no doubt that the saving resulting from the rapidity and completeness of the cures effected by good nursing, will be a considerable set-off against the increased cost of the nursing staff; though your Committee can offer no decided opinion as to the probable extent of the saving so effected.

2. Your Committee believe that accommodation equal at least, if not superior, to that afforded to the nurses in the London hospitals, can be provided in the Workhouse at a moderate outlay. It is estimated that, for the male hospital, a sum of from 400*l.* to 500*l.* would suffice to provide the rooms and to furnish them.

3. With reference to the supply of suitable nurses, your

Committee have to report that, as the authorities of the Nightingale Training School for nurses have offered to render to the Select Vestry all the assistance in their power in obtaining trained nurses, no great difficulty on this point need be apprehended. Were your Committee as sanguine as some of the hospital authorities whom they have consulted, as to the happy results to be expected from the introduction of trained nurses into the Workhouse, they would at once, with the utmost confidence, recommend that the whole of the hospital should, at the cost of the parish, be supplied with this class of officers; but, looking upon it as they do, as an experiment (at least in its economical results), they unanimously recommend that the system should, in the first instance, be tried in the male hospital

J. W. CROPPER,
Chairman.

The report of the Sub-Committee met with the approval of the Vestry. Some delay in the adoption of its recommendations was caused by a severe outbreak of fever in the town, which for the time absorbed all the resources of the Vestry and its officers. But on the 18th of May, 1865, a Lady Superintendent who had received a thorough training at Kaiserswerth and St. Thomas's, twelve Nightingale nurses from St. Thomas's, eighteen probationers, and fifty-two of the old pauper nurses were placed in charge of the patients in the male wards of the Workhouse Infirmary. By the judicious management of Mr. Carr, the most admirable arrangements were made for the accommodation of the nurses. Each superior nurse had a little room to herself, and the ex-pauper nurses were entirely separated from the other inmates of the Workhouse. It was hoped that by taking the best of the able-bodied inmates, separating them from the other paupers, and paying them small wages (say 5*l.* a year) they might be made available as assistant nurses, and that many of them might be elevated into independence and usefulness. It will be seen from the foregoing report of the Governor, that he always distrusted this part of the plan adopted; and after the system had been at work a year, this attempt to utilize pauper nurses in a workhouse hospital was found to have utterly failed. It was proved that in a town like Liverpool, with very few exceptions, those able-bodied women only become inmates of the Workhouse who are either tainted in character, or are exceptionally ill-educated and inefficient. The experiment, however, was not wholly useless. It conclusively established two facts: that such women are utterly unfit to be trusted as nurses; and that their employment in that capacity does not effect all the saving that might be supposed. It might be thought that the choice lay between such employment and maintaining the pauper in idleness, while paying a nurse in her stead. But it was found—as the Governor had always predicted—that when sent back from the hospital to the able-bodied wards, nearly the whole of these women left the Workhouse, and relieved the parish from the charge of their maintenance. Many of these women, when employed as nurses, remain in the Workhouse for the sake of what they can pick up or extort. And moreover, when they left it, the training they had received, such as it was, rendered them more intelligent, and perhaps not more unreliable nurses than those usually employed by the poor. It is not unlikely that in country places the unfitness of able-bodied paupers to become assistant nurses may be far less than it has been found to be in a great seaport town like Liverpool. They may probably be less universally tainted in character, and after a year or two of employment as under-nurses they may be able to maintain themselves in that capacity out-of-doors, thus not only relieving the parish of their own maintenance, but assisting to diminish sickness and pauperism among their neighbours. The point is one which must be left to local knowledge and experience. It might be well, however, not to promise them payment till after some length of probationary service. It was always after pay-day that the ex-pauper nurses were most liable to get drunk and misbehave. With the exception of the failure of the nurses taken from the pauper class, the first year's trial was sufficiently successful to induce a continuance of the experiment. It was impossible, however, to judge the result by statistics. None that were available could be considered as an evidence of success or failure, for several reasons. The season was very unhealthy, and to relieve the pressure on the space and resources of the hospital, steps were taken to treat slight cases outside, as will be seen from the following extract from the Minutes of the Finance Committee, 24th November, 1865:—

"The district medical officers, Dr. Gee, Mr. Barnes, and the Governor of the workhouse being in attendance, pursuant to resolution of the Workhouse Committee at its meeting yesterday, the practicability of limiting the admissions to the Workhouse Hospital was considered, and the district medical officers were requested to co-operate with the relieving officers in limiting such admissions to those cases that cannot be properly treated outside the Workhouse."

The endeavour to limit the admissions to serious cases would of course affect the returns, both as regards the time taken in curing, and the proportion of deaths. Even had there been no exceptional disturbing element, there is a defect in the statistics of workhouse hospitals which affects all inferences from them, in the absence of any careful classified list of cases kept by the medical officers, such as might fairly enable one to form a judgment from mere statistical tables. These, then, are not reliable as means of judgment, unless extending over a long period. The character of seasons, and nature of cases admitted, varies so much from year to year as to invalidate any deductions, unless founded on plete and minutely kept medical records. The following extracts, however, from the reports of the Governor, and the surgical and medical officers of the Workhouse, bear decisive witness to the value of the "new system," especially as contrasted with the "old system," which in 1865-66 still prevailed in the female wards. All these reports bear emphatic testimony to the merits and devotion of the Lady Superintendent and her staff. The medical men, it is noteworthy, speak strongly of the better discipline and far greater obedience to their orders observable where the trained nurses are employed—a point the more important because it is that on which, before experience has reassured them, medical and other authorities have often been most doubtful.

From the Report of the Governor.

Thursday, May 10, 1866.

The main feature in the new system of nursing consists in the superseding of pauper nurses, and appointing in their places competent trained nurses from the Nightingale School. These latter to have the assistance of "probationary nurses," or in other words, women of intelligence and of good character desirous of entering upon the duties of nursing the sick as a profession. A third class was also created, designated "Assistants." These were selected from the old pauper nurses, and it was decided that they should be paid, clothed, and receive rations equal in quality and quantity to those issued to the officers of the workhouse. The nurses, probationers, and assistants were placed under the control of a "Lady Superintendent," who was empowered to employ them in the manner to her seeming best for the proper care of the sick.

The Committee will be prepared to hear that the change was immediately followed by the most marked improvement in every respect. The most casual observer could not avoid perceiving it. This applies not only to the state of the wards, the care of the sick, but is particularly observable in the demeanour of the patients, upon whom the humanizing influences of a body of women of character, devotedly discharging their duties, has produced evident fruits.

The question has often been asked whether the "new system is likely to succeed?" The "old system" meant nothing more than this, that old, ignorant, and unreliable pauper women, many of whom were of doubtful character, were entrusted with the discharge, without pay, of responsible duties. These have been displaced, and active, intelligent, reliable women, trained and skilled as nurses, with good characters and pay, have been appointed to supersede them. It would be a great discredit if these latter did not discharge their duties incomparably better than the former could do. That they do so I am happy to be in a position to testify.

In the opening paragraph of this report it is stated that "assistant nurses" were appointed and placed upon pay from the ranks of the paupers. This I was always opposed to. Their employment has resulted in complete failure, as the following figures will prove. The total number appointed to this date is 141. Of these sixty-seven have been dismissed through drunkenness and other misconduct, and sixteen have resigned; while it is positively true that there is not one of the whole number to whom I could entrust the duties of serving out wine or other stimulants, or, in fact, any duty requiring the exercise of integrity.

The experience of the past year renders it certain that the Poor Law, as now existing, offers no impediments to the successful working out of the most complete scheme for the efficient nursing of the sick, in the manner advocated by the best friends of hospital nursing.

(*Signed*)
GEO. CARR.

From the Report of
Robert Gee, Esq. M.D. Physician to
the Workhouse Hospital.

5, Abercromby Square, Liverpool,
May 10, 1866.

Sir,

In the medical wards of a general hospital the cases vary so much in nature and degree from year to year, as to render it impossible to give a reliable statistical comparison of the value of a paid as distinguished from an unpaid staff of nurses. I am, therefore, necessarily compelled to report in general terms on the nursing of the last ten months in the male medical wards; premising that what I say in approbation of the new system, and the new staff of nurses must not be construed as an unfavourable reflection on the *whole* of the previous staff. The paid superintending nurses of departments, and a few of the unpaid pauper nurses, deserve great credit for their conduct, though their qualifications for the service were decidedly inferior to those of the trained "Nightingale" staff.

With regard to the latter I can cordially bear testimony to their ability, and to their unwearied and uniformly kind attention to the patients under their charge. As to their nursing in its specific sense, I may state my belief that in every case my directions and those of the House Surgeons have been rigidly carried out. The medicines, stimulants, &c. &c. have been carefully administered, and the other numerous but less agreeable duties have been faithfully and efficiently attended to. Under their charge I have perceived a marked improvement in the demeanour of the patients—in fact, the discipline of the wards is completely changed. There has been no disorder or irregularity, but a sense of comfort, order, and quiet pervades the whole department. I believe further, that every patient leaving the wards has been more or less morally elevated during his location there.

From the report of J. H. Barnes, Esq., Surgeon.

March 21, 1866.

Since my connection with the hospital last August we have had somewhat approaching a hundred operations, many of them of a serious and dangerous character, requiring not only prompt assistance at the time, but most persevering attention night and day for a long time after. Almost all these operations have been in the male hospital, and I have no hesitation in saying that what success has attended them has been greatly owing to the most efficient assistance rendered by the trained nurses; and from my experience of the assistance received from the pauper nurses, in the few cases of operation performed in the female hospital, I should feel great diffidence in undertaking on that side such operations as I have had on the other side: indeed on one or two occasions the pauper nurses ran away, and when induced to assist were so nervous and frightened as to be of little service.

Without any wish to speak harshly of the unpaid nurses employed on the female side of the hospital (who, I believe, strive to do their best, more especially since a feeling of emulation has been set up by the introduction of the paid trained nurses, of whom they are jealous), I am compelled to state my conviction that on that side my directions are not carried out with that necessary promptitude and skill that they are on the other side, and that in all I do there I feel as if I were working with blunted instruments. There is no want of inclination, but simply a want of ability. That *integrity of disposition, promptitude of action, tact in manipulation, gentleness of demeanour and kindly consideration* necessary to make a nurse are not found, or *to be* found in the inmates of a workhouse, and no amount of education can work out of them what never was in them. Almost always obtuse, and too often unprincipled, as a class they are thoroughly unreliable and quite unfitted to take charge of the sick and helpless, or the stimulants necessary for them. On this last point I have been informed by a former resident surgeon that he has known the pauper nurses appropriate the patient's stimulants, or withhold giving to a dying patient that ordered for him, that they might take it themselves after his death. It is difficult to bring home and prove these things, and I do not wish to say they now occur, but if we wish to put such conduct out of the region of possibility it can only be done by the employment of persons superior to the temptation so to act.

Persons of one class, as a rule, favour their own class, and there is a far better chance of double-dealers being detected when under the observation and care of a trained nurse, than when under the care of one of themselves. That such is the case my own experience testifies.

As far, therefore, as my experience extends of the system of trained nurses, whether regarding the saving of life, the restoration to health, or the relief of the suffering, it has been an undoubted success.

These reports were duly considered by the authorities; and after some discussion, it was resolved entirely to discontinue, in the male hospital ward, the employment of paupers as assistant nurses, and to substitute an additional number of probationers. A Sub-Committee of the Workhouse Committee was appointed to superintend and report upon the working of the system. These gentlemen devoted much time and attention to the subject, and at the close of the year undertook a minute inquiry into the operation of the old and new systems; examining personally the various officers of the Workhouse, from the Governor down to the pauper nurses in the female wards. Increased experience brought out in a yet stronger light the superior advantages of the employment of trained nurses. The very able, clear, and conclusive report of the Sub-Committee leaves little more to be said on the subject. It determined the Vestry to adopt the system in permanence, and to extend it to the whole of the Workhouse Infirmary, a year before the period fixed for the trial of the experiment had expired. It will be seen that the report of the second year's experience has a peculiar value, as bearing on the question whether, or how far, women may be competent to undertake one of the most delicate and difficult kinds of feminine work—one requiring special knowledge as well as special habits of punctual regularity, obedience, and thoughtfulness—without receiving any special training or education for such a duty. If the reforms about to be introduced into the pauper hospitals in London and elsewhere are not to end in failure and disappointment, provision must be made for training the nurses to be employed there, either before they enter the hospitals or within them. The report of the Sub-Committee of Superintendence is as follows:—

The Special Committee on Nursing, pursuant to resolution of the Workhouse Committee of the 7th of March instant, report,

That the Men's Hospital (exclusive of fever patients) is at present exclusively nursed by skilled, *i. e.* specially trained nurses and paid assistants, who are themselves undergoing training as nurses; the staff consisting of the Superintendent, nine of the nurses originally sent from the Nightingale School, five nurses who have been trained in the Workhouse, and fifteen probationary or assistant nurses.

Of the character of the nursing in this portion of the Workhouse, your Committee have heard but one opinion. The Governor and the Medical Officers concur in speaking of it in terms of the highest praise, and throughout the whole period during which the Committee have superintended it, no single circumstance has come to their knowledge calculated to make them speak of it otherwise than in terms of approval.

The nursing of the women's wards continues to be done by paupers under the superintendence of paid officers. The superintendence of these officers is of necessity very imperfect, as not only has each charge of from 150 to 200 patients, but these patients are located in several rooms, each ward containing about twenty patients. The only portion of the nursing, properly so called, which these officers undertake, is the administration of stimulants and in some exceptional cases of medicine. The bulk of it, as the giving of medicine, the dressing of wounds, the distribution of food, is left to be done by paupers. So much has from time to time been said of the untrustworthiness of pauper nurses, of the evils resulting to those patients who are placed exclusively under them, of the mischievous consequences upon the discipline of the Workhouse of a large number of petty offices being filled by able-bodied women, that your Committee believe they rightly interpret the feeling of the Select Vestry, as they undoubtedly do that of the general public, in supposing that the actual nursing of the sick in the Liverpool Workhouse can no longer be left in the hands of pauper nurses.

Starting from this point, your Committee considered that they had principally to inquire what sort of nursing can be most advantageously substituted for that of nursing by paupers. Two courses only appeared to be open to them—either to increase the number of paid officers, giving to each such a number of patients as she could reasonably be expected to look after, and treating each as an independent officer; or to extend over the whole hospital the system now in existence in the men's wards. Your Committee were much aided in forming a judgment upon this point, by what has taken place during the last few months in the fever hospital.

Here, originally, the paid attendants were in precisely the same position, with precisely similar duties as the paid officers in the women's hospital; but the number of patients rapidly diminishing, and no corresponding reduction taking place in the number of officers, the staff was so large that Dr. Gee felt able to call upon the officers to act as nurses. The result was what might have been anticipated, that although an improvement upon the old system of nursing by paupers was perceptible, the state of the nursing was still far short of the standard reached in the men's wards.

The officers were told to nurse, and they did their best, but never having themselves been taught, their attempts in a great measure failed; they were paid and retained as nurses, without being efficient nurses.

Committee therefore recommend that as soon as the requisite number of trained nurses can be procured, the nursing in the women's hospital, and afterwards in the fever hospital, be placed in the hands of trained and skilled nurses, acting under the direction and control of Miss Jones, the present Superintendent. The expenses (beyond the item of wages) attendant upon the necessary increase in the number of nurses will not be great, as all that will be necessary will be to convert two of the rooms now used for sick boys into sleeping apartments for the nurses. In making this recommendation, the Committee are glad to know that they are fortified by the unanimous opinion of the Governor and the Medical Officers of the Workhouse.

Your Committee are bound to add that they can produce no statistics shewing that the nursing in the men's hospital has been of any economical advantage to the Parish; but as it needs no argument to prove that the cheapest course that can be taken with a sick pauper is to cure him as quickly as possible; as it is evident that the care and attention of a skilled nurse must tend to a more speedy recovery; as the order and discipline of a well-regulated ward is more distasteful to many of the more worthless inmates, than the laxer management of a room in the hands of a pauper nurse; and as the abolition of a large number of petty offices for able-bodied paupers must lead to many of them leaving the Workhouse, there are strong grounds for hoping that the economical results of the change cannot but be beneficial.

With regard to the future, your Committee recommend that the Department of Nursing should be placed under the direction of a small committee of your body, and that all changes in the staff should be made only by them. From information they have received, your Committee have reason to believe that if, after the Workhouse is supplied with Nurses, the two classes of nurses, *i.e.* trained nurses and probationers, be maintained, the cost of the Department may be considerably lessened by training nurses for other hospitals; the cost of the probationers being either paid for by a Government grant, or by the bodies for whom the nurses may be trained.

THOMAS H. SATCHELL,
RICHARD BRIGHT,
THOMAS OWEN.

March 15, 1867.

This report was unanimously adopted by the Workhouse Committee and by the Vestry; and already the new system has been extended to the Female Wards. It is in contemplation to extend it also to the Fever Hospital, as soon as a sufficient number of suitable nurses shall have been trained.

It will be observed that the report contemplates the training of probationers for other Workhouse Infirmaries. And it is, indeed, to be hoped that in this and other ways the Liverpool Workhouse Hospital may serve as a normal school, from which the system there adopted may spread. The *special* expenses of such a school would naturally be borne by the parishes which profited by its services in educating nurses for them, or by the Government. But this point is one which, as yet, has hardly demanded practical consideration.

The experiment whose results have been recorded, could hardly have been tried at all—certainly could not have achieved such rapid success—had it not been for the powerful and liberal assistance of Miss Nightingale, and the Trustees of the Nightingale Fund. Feeling how very important was the extension of the system of superior professional nursing, now gradually gaining ground in general hospitals, to workhouses, they sent, to assist in the initial experiment made in this direction, a lady superintendent and twelve superior nurses—a very expensive and quite invaluable contribution. To the Liverpool Vestry and its officers belongs the credit of having overcome all the difficulties, and persevered in spite of all the discouraging incidents, which necessarily attended an attempt to introduce a new system of management into such an institution as a Workhouse Hospital, combining as it does two subjects so different in their aspects and conditions of treatment, so difficult to deal with together, as pauperism and sickness. Of the Lady Superintendent I shall say little. When a lady leaves a happy home, and goes through a long and laborious course of training to fit herself for such a situation, purely because, feeling that she possessed the capacity for nursing, and the requisite health, energy, strength, and spirits, she desired to devote such powers to the service of those who stood most in need of them, human praise or criticism of her choice is out of place. One of the incidental results of her exertions has to her, no doubt, been even a higher reward than that improvement in the condition of the sick, in their progress towards recovery, and their material comfort, which has been the direct object of her labours. The improvement in the tone and behaviour of the patients has been wonderful. Many of the inmates of a pauper hospital are persons of the worst character, and its wards, under the control of pauper nurses, often present scenes so disgusting that the respectable poor shrink from them with utter abhorrence, and after once becoming acquainted with them, will often rather die than return thither. When the trained nurses were first introduced, the most offensive language was frequently heard in the wards; and the Lady Superintendent has repeatedly been obliged to call upon the Governor two or three times during one Sunday to use his authority to put a stop to actual fighting. Now, though his support is always promptly rendered, she is rarely compelled to apply for it; the feeling of the wards promptly suppresses all offensive language or unseemly behaviour in the presence of the nurses. The following letter from Sir H. Verney, Chairman of the Nightingale Committee, serves to illustrate the influence of the nurses upon the conduct of the patients; he came down to Liverpool to inspect the Hospital, and ascertain the progress of the work:—

Liverpool, October 3, 1866.

My dear Sir,

By the kindness of Mr. Carr I have paid a visit to the Workhouse, and have been greatly interested by remarking the change among the male pauper sick, effected since I was here about two years since. I conclude that this is owing to the nursing by a class of females so entirely different to those who nursed the male paupers at that time, and who still nurse the female sick. I have always seen that the influence of respectable and well-educated females over the most debased men is very striking. Men of that character, accustomed to intercourse with only degraded women, feel the restraining and humanizing power of virtuous and well-mannered females. They have never been admitted into intercourse with such before, and they are most beneficially affected by it. I have been told that the police officers, who sometimes come to the Workhouse on business, and who see the sick paupers, are much astonished. They see the men whom they have known as the very worst characters, conducting themselves with propriety and decency, and giving no cause of complaint.

I am sure that the Workhouse Committee must rejoice and feel thankful that there is such a change in the condition of the poor creatures brought under their rule.

Miss Jones, and her nurses and probationers, must have had much difficulty at first—indeed their work is still very trying; but the improved demeanour of the men must be highly gratifying and encouraging to them. I walked through the female sick wards; they were clean and sweet, but I could not help contrasting the pauper nurses who attended them, with the intelligent-looking respectable attendants of the men.

I thank you for the note of introduction which procured admission for me, and

I am, Yours very faithfully,

HARRY VERNEY.

Such, and so entirely satisfactory to the Guardians, were the results of the experiment of nursing by trained nurses, as tried for two years in the Male Wards of the Liverpool Workhouse Infirmary. It is in order to render those results, the experience acquired in this initiatory attempt, available for the assistance and encouragement of others, that they have been thus briefly recorded. Much more might have been said; but what is here set down is sufficient to explain all that practical men would wish to know, and it would be presumption to waste the time of such men with comments and inferences which they are perfectly able to make for themselves.

One suggestion, in conclusion, I may be permitted to offer. In all unions or parishes where additional accommodation may be required, whether for patients or for healthy paupers, it is eminently desirable that in providing it regard should be had to the entire separation, at once or at a future time, of the sick and infirm from the able-bodied, as will be the case, at least partially, under the new régime introduced in the Metropolis by Mr. Gathorne Hardy's Bill. Miss Nightingale has from the first held and expressed a strong opinion in favour of the separation of the hospital and workhouse administrations. The Governor of the Liverpool Workhouse, Mr. Carr, expressed himself decidedly in the same sense; and the Chairman of the Workhouse Committee and of the Sub-Committee appointed to superintend the Hospital, has been induced by practical experience warmly to advocate the absolute separation of the Workhouse and the Infirmary. So large a proportion of the able-bodied inmates of the workhouse are drunken, lazy, and vicious, that, if the poor-law relief is not to become a temptation and an injury to the honest and struggling poor, the discipline must be almost of a penal character. The paramount object must be to make the workhouse, if not absolutely unpleasant, less agreeable than the condition of laborious and striving poverty. On the other hand, in a hospital the paramount and almost the only object is to promote recovery and to mitigate suffering; all other considerations yield to this, and consequently the treatment must necessarily be liberal in spirit and indulgent in fact. The modes of treatment necessary for the good management of the hospital patient and of the able-bodied pauper, respectively, are distinct—almost opposite: the infirmary and the workhouse must be controlled on divergent, and even contrary principles; and by bringing the two together under one roof and one administration, they injure each other. The indulgence of the infirmary creeps into the workhouse, or the sternness of workhouse rules cripples the benevolent energy which should rule the infirmary. And the treatment of the able-bodied pauper becomes too lax, or he is tempted to scheme, and does scheme, to get himself transferred to the more comfortable quarters close at hand; a desire so prevalent as to give rise to malingering—the wilful production of disease: while, partly no doubt in order to counteract this tendency, there is in such mixed establishments an unconscious disposition to treat the hospital patient with the same stern economy that is justly made the rule in dealing with able-bodied pauperism, but which, in the infirmary, is not only cruel, but in the long run is not truly economical. Another most serious evil is entailed upon the hospital by connexion with the workhouse. The habits and traditions prevalent among the habitual paupers—able-bodied paupers—in the workhouse (at least in the workhouse of a large town), are too often deeply infected with cunning, deception, and dishonesty of all sorts, against which strict precaution and stern repression are requisite; and it is most important that no communication should be allowed, whereby these habits of vice and stratagem might be introduced into the hospital, where indulgence is the rule, and where many things strictly denied to the inmates of the workhouse, as stimulants for instance, are necessarily permitted. The introduction of workhouse tricks into a hospital, where they cannot be met by workhouse control, must bring in an element of confusion, disorder, and waste, and therefore the intercommunication which might introduce those tricks should be as effectually prevented as possible, which it cannot be while the two institutions are, as at present, combined. The two systems—to use an English word in its French sense—demoralize each other; and even in the English sense, their union demoralizes the individuals subject to each.

When this is better understood and more clearly apprehended, as it soon will be, through the experience of several Unions in which the separation has been already resolved on—it is probable that it will be enforced by law. This may be expected to take place in no very long time; and then it will be found that any expenditure incurred in providing increased accommodation on a plan which does not recognise the necessity of separation has been, in part at least, thrown away; and the work will have to be done, and the money to be spent, over again.

ARMY SANITARY ADMINISTRATION, AND ITS REFORM UNDER THE LATE LORD HERBERT.

Read by Florence Nightingale at the London Meeting of the "Congrès de Bienfaisance," June, 1862.

It has been well and truly said that, in long wars, the real arbiter of the destinies of nations is not the sword, but pestilence.

It is this destroying angel which, following on the march of armies, exacts of every man to the full whatever penalties follow on the infraction of natural law.

In times past, war has been conducted in more or less forgetfulness, sometimes in total oblivion, of the fact, that the soldier is a mortal man, subject to all the ills following on wet and cold, want of shelter, bad food, excessive fatigue, bad water, intemperate habits, and foul air.

And so the waste of human life, and the destruction of human health and happiness, have been, in all ages, many times greater from disease than from actual encounter in the field.

If peace has its victories as well as war, it has also its unnecessary losses from disease and death. Only the losses of peace are greater than those of war; because they are daily and constant, while war occurs at intervals of time.

To endeavour to prevent this destruction of life is by no means to encourage war, no more than to attend on the sick and wounded in a field hospital is to encourage war.

The object is primarily one of humanity. It is to save life, and to diminish suffering. And all who engage in this work are, in the best sense, savers of men.

Highest among such must be ranked Sidney Herbert.

As years pass on, so will the work, which he was a main agent in accomplishing, become better known and followed up.

And who can tell how much systematic attempts, made by all nations to diminish the horrors of this great curse, war, may not lead the way to its total disappearance from the earth?

The faithful records of all wars are records of preventible suffering, disease, and death. It is needless to illustrate this truth, for we all know it. But it is only from our latest sorrow, the Crimean catastrophe, that dates the rise of army sanitary administration in this country.

The losses then incurred, and the experience derived from these, induced her Majesty to issue the now famous royal commission on the "Sanitary State of the Army," composed of men qualified to grapple with the whole subject, and to suggest the necessary remedies. Sidney Herbert presided over that commission, and embodied its results in a masterly report, shoeing, for the first time, the great and unnecessary mortality to which the army was at all times subject, the diseases occasioning it, their removable causes, and the administrative reforms required to arrest this awful loss of life and efficiency. At that time, the death rate among soldiers from consumption and tubercular diseases *alone* (the monstrous products of breathing foul air), exceeded the *total* death *from all causes* among the civil population of the corresponding ages. The total mortality in the army was nearly double—in the Guards more than double—that of the civil population. It is now actually *less* than in civil life.

Sidney Herbert's report laid the foundation of army sanitary reform. Lord Panmure, aware of its price, issued, under Sidney Herbert's advice, four sub-commissions for giving effect to its recommendations:—

One, the Barrack and Hospital Improvement Commission, examined the barracks and military hospitals of the united kingdom, and found their sanitary condition as to overcrowding, want of ventilation, want of drainage, imperfect water supply, &c., sufficient to account for most of the excessive death rate from which the troops occupying them had suffered. These establishments have, under the direction of the commission, been provided with combined ventilation and warming, without machinery of any kind. Drainage has been introduced, or improved. Water supply has been extended, baths introduced both for barracks and hospitals, and the lavatory arrangements generally improved. The barrack kitchens have been completely remodelled; the wasteful cooking apparatus, only fit for boiling, has been replaced by improved and economical cooking ranges for roasting, &c., so that the men may now have the change of cookery required for health, instead of the eternal soup and boiled beef. Gas has been introduced into many barracks, instead of the couple of "dips," which only made the barrack room look darker still, and by the light of which it was impossible for the men to read, or to pursue any occupation except smoking. Many important structural alterations for increasing window light, circulating fresh air by removing useless partitions, for ventilating stables, abolishing ash-pits, &c., have been carried out. More simple and healthy principles for the construction of future barracks and hospitals, for ensuring better drainage, efficient ventilation, more cubic space for both sick and well, and greater facilities for administration and discipline, have been laid down, and applied in several new structures;—amongst others, in the great "Herbert Hospital" at Woolwich.

The labours of the same commission have since been extended to the Mediterranean stations, where they were greatly required; and, it is to be hoped, will be farther extended to the West Indies and Canada.

The result of the improvements, already made, is that just one half of the Englishmen that enter the army die (at home stations) as formerly died.

The *total mortality* at home stations, *from all diseases*, is now actually *less* (by above one per thousand per annum) than was formerly the mortality from consumption and chest diseases *alone*. The reduction in deaths from consumption has been as remarkable: in some arms one-half, in others two-thirds of the mortality from this fatal disease has disappeared.

To shew what has already been done, I have transferred, from the Report of the Royal Commission, a diagram, shewing the death statistics of the English male population, between the ages of fifteen and forty-five, and the death statistics of the infantry of the line, serving at home, from 1837 to 1846. This is how Sidney Herbert found the army. I have added a third division, shewing the death rate of the same infantry for the three years following the introduction of sanitary improvement, 1859-60-61. This is how Sidney Herbert left the army.

As a supplement to the improvements in barrack cook-houses (already referred to), Lord Herbert directed a school for practical cookery to be established at Aldershot, for the training of regimental and hospital cooks; instead of taking it for granted, as was the practice, that any man could cook just as he could mount guard. This school is gradually supplying both regiments and hospitals with cooks capable of giving men a wholesome meal.

The second sub-commission was appointed for re-organizing the New Code of army medical department, and for framing a code of regulations for Regulations the hospital and sanitary service of the army. This commission found that, according to existing practice, no provision was made for systematically caring for the soldier's *health*, but only for his *sickness*. The chief recognised function of the army medical officer was attending men in hospital; but in no way was it considered his duty to render it unnecessary for men to come into hospital at all.

To supply this great want, the commission drew up a code for introducing the sanitary element (for the first time) into the army, defining the positions of commanding and medical officers, and their relative duties and responsibilities regarding the soldier's health, constituting the regimental surgeon the sanitary adviser of his commanding officer, who is now bound to give effect to all sanitary recommendations made by his medical officer, unless he can assign satisfactory reasons *in writing* to the superior authority for non-compliance.

The same code contains regulations for organizing general hospitals, and for improving the administration of regimental hospitals, both in peace and during war. Formerly, general hospitals in the field had to be improvised, on no defined principles, and on no defined personal responsibility. The wonder is, not that they broke down, as they did in all our wars, but that they could be made to stand at all. In all our wars our general hospitals have been signal failures, fatal examples of how to kill, not to cure. All this is now changed; and, with the most ordinary administrative capacity, the sick during war may now have every necessary care and comfort.

This code is the best ever framed; and, in practice, has been found to succeed in every climate, whether at home, in garrison, or in the field. It has been successfully tested in two expeditions, since issued by Lord Herbert in 1859. On the day which took him from us, its general hospital system was realized in the hospital at Woolwich, including its governor, principal medical officer, captain of orderlies, female nurses, and their female superintendent, &c., which system will be transferred to the magnificent hospital, now being built there, of which Lord Herbert was the founder, and which will bear his name. He also directed a plan to be drawn up for the organization of a second general hospital at Devonport, on the same principles, which will shortly be carried into effect.

The third sub-commission was charged with organizing a practical school at Chatham, for instructing candidates for army medical service in military hygiene and other specialities.

Formerly young men were sent to attend sick and wounded soldiers, who *perhaps* had never dressed a serious wound, or never attended a bedside, except in the midst of a crowd of students, following in the wake of some eminent lecturer—who *certainly* had never been instructed in the most ordinary sanitary knowledge; although one of their most important functions was hereafter to be the prevention of disease in climates, and under circumstances where *prevention* is everything, and medical treatment often little or nothing.

The sub-commission drew up an admirable scheme; and the school at Chatham was opened by Sidney Herbert in person, in 1860. Already its results have been most satisfactory. A large number of men of high attainments have been sent from it into the army; and we may confidently expect a lower sick rate and death rate (especially on foreign stations and on field service) as one of its results, as well as higher hospital efficiency.

The fourth sub-commission was charged with the duty of re-organizing the army medical statistics, which were then in such a condition as to afford very incomplete data, especially during war. These statistics have been reformed, and are now by far the best and most useful in Europe. They can be reduced with much less labour, and with much greater promptitude than formerly; because the manner of recording cases is now much more precise, and there is a special division in the army medical department for reducing them to obtain the results; while they enable the exact state of health, of every regiment and station, to be ascertained, and any unusual amount of disease, *with its removable causes*, to be brought at once to the cognizance of the authorities.

In the course of years they will add immensely to our knowledge of army diseases, as well as of those incident to particular climates and seasons.

Although the first annual report under the new system, being a *first* report, does not give all the data, regimental and stational, required by the instructions, yet every succeeding year's experience will render these annual reports more complete and more valuable.

Of all these commissions Sidney Herbert was head and centre. He superintended himself carefully every step of their procedure, and took his share of the work, as well as the responsibility attaching to it in his public capacity, by identifying himself with the reforms. In England it is so much the custom to look upon statesmen merely in their political, and not in their administrative capacity, that it is almost forgotten that they have an administrative function at all. No one thinks of a secretary of state, *e. g.*, as the head of an office which has in its hands the lives and morals of men. But Sidney Herbert, although his passion, his hereditary occupation, to which he was born and bred, was politics, yet made his administrative labours greater, set his administrative object higher, recoiled from none of its dry fatigues, and attained its highest usefulness. What has been well-advised to a rising statesman, he performed. He did not sink in politics the powers which were meant for mankind.

Army medical officers had felt much and just dissatisfaction with their position in the army. The royal commission advised therefore the preparation of another warrant, ensuring to these officers the rank and emolument to which their services entitled them. It was framed by Sidney Herbert, and issued by General Peel in 1858.

Another great reform was introduced into the Purveying Department, which, like many others, had no well-defined position, duties, or responsibilities. It was efficient or inefficient almost by chance. Like other departments, it broke down when tried by war; and all its defects were visited on the sick and wounded men, for whose special benefit it professed to exist.

To put an end to this, and to introduce method into the service. Lord Herbert issued in 1861 a new purveyor's code and regulations, re-organizing the department in accordance with the views expressed by himself, as Chairman of the Royal Commission. The regulations now define with precision the duties of each class of purveyor's officers, together with their relation to the army medical department. They provide all necessaries and comforts for men in hospital (both in the field and at home) on fixed scales; instead of requiring sick and wounded men (even in the field) to bring with them into hospital articles for their own use, and which they had lost before reaching it, These regulations have been already tried, both for home and field service, and have been found to answer every purpose.

Lord Herbert also named a committee to re-organize the army hospital corps. In former times there were no proper attendants on the sick. For regimental hospitals a steady man was appointed hospital sergeant, and two or three soldiers, fit for nothing else, were sent into the hospital, to be under the orders of the medical officer; who, if he were fortunate enough to find one man fit to nurse a patient, was sure to lose him by his being recalled "to duty;" sometimes, indeed, men were mounted in rotation over sick in hospital as they would mount guard over a store. And this is still done in India, and in some regiments at home.

No special training was considered necessary; no one, except the medical officer, who was helpless, had the least idea that attendance on the sick is as much a special business as medical treatment.

Unsuccessful attempts had been made to organize a corps of orderlies, unconnected with regiments: the result was most unsatisfactory. Lord Herbert's committee proposed to constitute a corps—the members of which, for regimental purposes, are to be carefully selected by the commanding and medical officers—specially trained for their duties, and then attached permanently to the regimental hospital, from which they cannot be removed to the ranks, except for proved incapacity or breach of discipline. This was carried into effect shortly after his death.

The crowning testimony of the great national importance of the new system of sanitary administration, inaugurated by Lord Herbert, is to be found in the last Chinese expedition, where his reforms were first practically tested. An expeditionary force was sent to the opposite side of the world, into a hostile country, notorious for its epidemic diseases. Every required arrangement for the preservation of health was made, with the result that the mortality of this force, including wounded, was little more than three per cent. per annum, while the "constantly sick" in hospital were about the same as at home. Let us contrast with this great success what happened during a former war in China. The 26th Cameronians, a "total abstinence" regiment, and one of the finest and most healthy in the British service, was landed at Chusan, 900 strong, and left to its fate without any sanitary care. In two months only twenty men could be got together.

To take another contrast upon a larger scale. During the first months of the Crimean war, from September 1854 to March 1855, the death rate among the British troops was sixty per cent. per annum, until means were taken to prevent this fearful sweep of death. During the same months, the "constantly sick" in the hospitals were sevenfold those in the war hospitals in China.

Impressed with the enormous death rate and loss of efficiency in the Indian army. Lord Herbert undertook in 1859 the presidency of Commission, the Royal Commission on the "sanitary state" of that army, called together to devise means for reducing these great losses. He was obliged to relinquish this to Lord Stanley in 1861, on account of official business, and, alas! of failing health. But by that time the evidence received from Indian stations had been sufficient to convince him that removable causes, of far greater importance and intensity than any which have been discovered in our home stations, were destroying the lives of our soldiers, and the physical efficiency of the Indian army.

Among other reforms initiated during Lord Herbert's life, but incomplete at his death, were the following:—

He had seen that the sanitary defects in barracks and hospitals had on arisen from the unsatisfactory manner in which these buildings had been planned and constructed. No one engaged on them had had any knowledge of the requirements for health. If they had been made to put guns and stores in, and not men at all, or horses, they could not, in fact, have been worse. There was no recognition of the necessity even of space, or of fresh air, or of drainage, either for sick or well. To prevent this in future, Lord Herbert called together a committee, to inquire into the present system of executing barrack works, and to suggest administrative improvements.

The department, charged with spending money on buildings to keep men healthy, knew little about the principles of healthy construction, such knowledge not having been required of them.

The result of the labours of the committee, it is expected, will be a better and more economical organization, a proper training in the principles of sanitary works, and a total change in the sanitary construction of our future military buildings.

Another very important commission was also called, to consider the question how best to provide soldiers' day-rooms and institutes, in order to struggle with the great moral evil supposed to be inseparable from garrisons and camps.

Lord Herbert saw that, at present, the soldier was hardly thought of as a man at all. The effect of moral agencies upon him was practically ignored. He (Lord Herbert) had taught every one, by this time, the results of treating the soldier physically as if he were not a human being, subject to the laws of physical health. And, in the moral tone of garrisons and camps, he recognised the legitimate results of treating the soldier morally, as if he were not under the laws of moral health. Placed, as he is, under strict restraint, lodged in a crowded, uncomfortable, barrack-room— without privacy, without social intercourse, except that afforded by the canteen or by some much worse place; without home ties; without occupation or amusement, except such as is provided for him by those (and they are everywhere) who pander to his passions—the soldier has a position most unfavourable to his moral nature. And just as the soldier was formerly accused of dying unnecessarily, or because it could not be helped, the real causes being all the while ignored; so now, the consequences of overlooking moral causes go by the name of "camp vices." Not that nothing has been done in the way of direct teaching to counteract the evil; but, all the while, the immoral agencies or temptations by which the man is surrounded, have been left untouched; while no counteracting agencies of a moral kind have been provided to cope with these.

In civil life at home, it is supposed inconsistent with individual liberty to put down bad places of resort, and to prevent open temptations to profligacy; while, in certain continental states, it is *not* supposed against liberty or morals to make prostitution as little disagreeable as possible—viz., by "regulating" it, to avert the consequences of this vice, leaving all the temptations just as they were.

Lately, the remedy alluded to has been repeatedly urged for Aldershot, in the face of the notorious fact that, while no proper places of resort or occupation have been created for the men, the remedy would leave the abominations of the town to go on untouched.

In dealing with this question, there are obvious principles. Governments *can* prevent this open infamous trading, as they do other open infamous trading. They *can* prevent open temptations to vice, as they can prevent open temptations to crime. They can do these things both for the civilian and the soldier. But for the soldier they can do more; and it is this which the committee on soldiers' day-rooms was called to consider by Lord Herbert.

They have shown that the men's barracks can be made more of a home—can be better provided with libraries and reading-rooms; that separate rooms can be attached to barracks where men can meet their comrades, sit with them, talk with them, have their newspaper and their coffee, if they want it, play innocent games, and write letters; that every barrack, in short, may easily be provided with a kind of soldiers' club, to which the men can resort when off duty, instead of to the everlasting barrack-room or the demoralizing dram-shop; and that, in large camps or garrisons, such as Aldershot and Portsmouth, the men may easily have a club of their own out of barracks.

The committee also recommended increased means of occupation, in the way of soldiers' workshops, outdoor games and amusements, and rational recreation by lectures and other means.

The plan has been tried with great success at Gibraltar, Chatham, Montreal. There is no reason why it should not succeed elsewhere. At all events, let it be tried.

Lord Herbert's latest act was directing an inquiry at Aldershot, as to the best means of introducing the system there. The country will support the cherished scheme of its dead statesman.

This is a short sketch of the labours and successes of Lord Herbert's last brief administration. The lesson which these reforms teach is, that the real foundation of War Office efficiency is to be laid in the efficient working of each department—in simplifying procedure, abolishing all divided responsibility, clearly defining the duties of each officer—in giving direct responsibility to each head of a department—and, lastly, in placing all the departmental heads in direct communication with the Secretary of State. It is by this procedure that the spirit which was breathed into Lord Herbert's reforms, may be expected to accomplish what *he* constantly kept before him as the great object of his official life—viz., to increase the efficiency, improve the position, and preserve the health of the British soldier.

There were indeed other important reforms made by Lord Herbert during this his last short tenure of office. But not for these, or so much for these as for the rest, will he be remembered. He will be remembered chiefly as the first war minister who ever seriously set himself to the task of saving life—who ever took the trouble to master a difficult subject so wisely and so well, as to be able himself, and to show the way to others, to husband the resources of this country, in which human life is of more value than in any other—of more value than any thing else.

To the army, in the person of Sir John Pringle, is due the credit of first having recognised the real, ever-operating effects of physical laws on human health and life. To the army, Sidney Herbert has, a century later, bequeathed the administrative means of applying those laws, so as to mitigate or to prevent the very diseases which previous administrators ignorantly supposed inseparable from the soldier's occupations.

The results cannot fail to re-act on the whole progress of sanitary reform in civil life. Let us hope that the great lesson which has been taught, will have its weight with those charged with the duty of protecting the public health.

HEALTH TEACHING IN TOWNS AND VILLAGES.

RURAL HYGIENE.

By Florence Nightingale, 1894

I have been pressed to write a paper, for the Leeds Conference of Women Workers, on Rural Health and Rural Health Missioners; and, though sorely entangled by pressing matters, I am the more anxious to do so because of the great attention which many ladies seem to be giving to the subject, and which appears to be spreading not only West but East. In two of the provinces of wide India it has been asked whether something could not be done there by instructed native Lecturers, who were also to *go round the village showing the people on the spot* where to put their refuse, how to keep their water-supply pure, &c., &c. And in one of these provinces the Lecturers were to be seconded by instructed native *women* visiting and teaching health habits to the village poor native *women in their own homes.* And the true word has been spoken: What can be done for the health of the *home* without the woman of the *home*?

Let not England lag behind—especially not in the conviction that nothing *can* be done without personal friendship with the women to be taught. It is a truism to say that the women who teach in India must know the languages, the religions, superstitions, and customs of the women to be taught in India. It ought to be a truism to say the very same for England. We must not talk *to* them, or *at* them, but *with* them.

A great man who has just passed away from us used to

advise his young men, when they entered life, to make personal acquaintance with the poor, whether they took or not to "works of philanthropy." He did not believe in any "philanthropy" which was not in fact what the word means—the love of men. But the knowledge of a man must go before the love for him— acquaintance, friendship, love can only come in this order; and the love that springs from the sympathy of a close and accurate knowledge of the ways, the habits, the lives of the poor is not a mere sentiment, but an active and a fruitful enthusiasm.

This is eminently the case with cottage mothers, in the matter of Rural Hygiene. You must know them, not as a class, but each one by herself, in order to do her service in this all-important matter.

And now I propose with your leave to touch upon—

1. The present machinery of Rural Public Health.
2. The present state of Rural Hygiene.
3. What the women have to do with it.
4. (In answer to many questions asked.) Some sketch of the scheme of Health-at-Home training and work.
5. What we mean by personal acquaintance and friendship between the women instructors and women to be instructed, always bearing in mind that the latter differ as widely from each other in character as they do in the circumstances of their lives

And to begin with:

1. What is the Existing Machinery of Public Health in what are called—with a grim sarcasm—our Rural *Sanitary* Districts? Is health or sickness, life or death, the greatest miracle in the present condition of things? To some of us the greatest miracle, repeated every day, is that we can live at all in the surroundings which our ignorance and neglect create.

There is the *Board of Guardians:* "Sanitary Authority," who give the tag-end of their time to a subject which might monopolise the whole of it, and yet not be exhausted.

Medical Officer of Health: generally a busy man with a private practice covering a very large area, who earns a pittance for doing a most important public duty; a man appointed to his office and maintained in it by those whom he ought to criticise fearlessly and openly, when they are careless about the health of those dependent on them. His salary, which ought to be proportionate to his capital of knowledge ever accumulating, and his income of experience rolling up as years go on, which should give him an opportunity for sufficient leisure to work at public health as a scientific study, apart from his medical practice—his salary, which should be enough for this, is often hardly sufficient for his necessary travelling expenses as a public official—sometimes only a few pounds per annum.

Sanitary Inspector: an official appointed by the Guardians, who are at liberty to select anyone they like, without any guarantee whatever that he has either the knowledge or the will to do his work, but upon the efficient performance of which may depend the health and even the lives of many hundred families in the district he inspects. He may be—sometimes has been— an unsuccessful farmer or tradesman, and he may be entirely independent of the control of the Medical Officer, who generally has had nothing whatever to do with his appointment, and is powerless to dismiss him.

We all know that in 1890 an Act was passed—there are more than 100 sections in it—for the Housing of the Working Classes. It is an Act which consolidates the wisdom and experience of experts, and was backed by the authority of the most influential men in the country. On paper there could hardly be a more perfect Health Directory for making our "Sanitary" Authorities and our "Sanitary" Districts worthy of the title they bear. We have everything defined for us that can require a definition. We have "powers" given to everyone who can possibly wish to have them. We have duties imposed upon our officials in language that is as clear and precise as the best draftsmen in England could make it.

We have awful threats launched against any and every dwelling-house which appears to a Medical Officer of Health "to be in a state

so dangerous or injurious to health as to be unfit for human habitation." In fact, everything is provided for, except the two things more necessary than all the rest, namely, the money to pay for and the will to carry out the reforms. And it is perfectly well known that, if this law were enforced immediately and completely, say, three-fourths of the rural districts in England would be depopulated, and we should have hundreds of thousands of houseless poor upon our hands, for such, at least, is the proportion of houses unfit for habitation in our rural districts.

We all know that, even where the law can and ought to be enforced, it is daily and persistently evaded to the great danger of public health—*e.g.* where Dairies, Cow-sheds, and Milk-shops Regulations are supposed to be in force, and where there is practically no registration; and no inspection exists that is worthy of the name.

These are the facts as they are.

Now let us consider *what they ought to be.*

We want independent Medical Officers of Health—appointed by the County Council, and removable only by them—men trained up for this as a profession; we want Sanitary Inspectors, with a proper qualification, appointed with the Medical Officer's approval; we want that each Medical Officer should be informed as to all approaches of dangerous disease, and bound in his turn to supply the information for other neighbouring districts; we want Sanitary Inspectors who are duly qualified by examination, acting under the directions of the Medical Officers, in order that they may feel themselves responsible for their appointment and co-operators in their work; Sanitary Inspectors who are not removable unless for neglect of duty, and certain to be removed if they do persistently neglect it.

We want a fully trained Nurse for every district, and a Health

Missioner. We want a *Water-supply* to each village, pure and plentiful; Rain-water properly stored; *Earth closets—Scavenging*: as necessary a public duty as paving and lighting; *Gardens* near houses, and allotments where refuse and privy contents are used for manure; *Cottage-owners* made amenable to sanitary laws, compelling the landlord to give his cottages the essentials for health as far as construction is concerned; *School* teaching of health rules, made interesting and clear by diagrams showing dangers of foul drains and so forth. [But we must not expect too much practical result from this. It has failed, except as a book or lesson, where it has been tried in India. The school-*master himself* should be a health apostle.] When our water is poisoned, we want to know it; then we shall avoid it. But it is far more difficult to get people to avoid poisoned air, for they drink it in by the gallon all night in their bedrooms, and too often in the day.

We will now deal with the

2. Present State of Rural Hygiene, which is indeed a pitiful and disgusting story, dreadful to tell.

For the sake of giving actual facts,—it is no use lecturing upon drainage, water-supply, wells, pig-sties, storage of excrement, storage of refuse, &c., &c., *in general*; they are dreadfully concrete,—I take leave to give the facts of one rural district, consisting of villages and one small market town, as described by a Local Government Board official this year; and I will ask the ladies here present whether they could not match these facts in every county in the kingdom. Perhaps, too, the lady lecturers on Rural Hygiene will favour us with some of their experiences.

A large number of the poor-cottages have been recently condemned as "unfit for human habitation," but though "unfit" many are still "inhabited," from lack of other accommodation.

Provision for conveying away surface and slop water is conspicuous either by its absence or defect. The slop-water stagnates and sinks into the soil all round the dwellings, aided by the droppings from the thatch. [It has been known that the bedroom slops are sometimes emptied out of window.] There *are* inside sinks, but the waste-pipe is often either untrapped or not disconnected.

It is a Government Official who says all this.

Water-supply almost entirely from shallow wells, often uncovered, mostly in the cottage garden, not far from a pervious privy pit, a pig-sty, or a huge collection of house refuse, polluted by the foulness soaking into it. The liquid manure from the pig-sty trickles through the ground into the well. Often after heavy rain the cottagers complain that their well-water becomes thick.

The water in many shallow wells has been analysed. And some have been closed; others *cleaned out*. But when no particular impurity is detected, no care has been taken to stop the too threatening pollution, or to prohibit the supply. In one village which *had* a pump, it was so far from one end that a pond in an adjoining field was used for their supply.

It may be said that, up to the present time, *practically* nothing has been done by the Sanitary Authorities to effect the removal of house refuse, &c.

In these days of investigation and statistics, where results are described with microscopic exactness and tabulated with mathematical accuracy, we seem to think figures will do instead of facts, and calculation instead of action. We remember the policeman who watched his burglar enter the house, and waited to make quite sure whether he was going to commit robbery with violence or without, before interfering with his operations. So as we read such an account as this we seem to be watching, not robbery, but murder going on, and to be waiting for the rates of mortality to go up before we interfere; we wait to see how many of the children playing round the houses shall be stricken down. We wait to see whether the filth will really trickle into the well, and whether the foul water really will poison the family, and how many will die of it. And then, when enough have died, we think it time to spend some money and some trouble to stop the murders going further, and we enter the results of our "masterly inactivity" neatly in tables; but we do not analyse and tabulate the saddened lives of those who remain, and the desolate homes in our "*sanitary*" "districts."

Storage of Excrement in these Villages.—This comes next. And it is so disgustingly inefficient that I write it on a separate sheet, to be omitted if desired. But we must remember that if we cannot bear with it, the national health has to bear with it, and especially the children's health. And I add, as a fact in another Rural District to the one quoted above, that, in rainy weather, the little children may play in the privy or in the so-called "barn" or small outhouse, where may be several privies, several pigs, and untold heaps of filth. And as the little faces are very near the ground, children's diarrhœa and diseases have been traced to this miasma.

Cess-pit privies.—The *cess-pits are excavations* in the ground; often left unlined. Sometimes the privy is a wooden sentry-box, placed so that the fœcal matter falls directly into a ditch. Cess-pits often very imperfectly or not at all covered. Some privies with a cubic capacity of 18 or 20 feet are emptied from once to thrice yearly. But we are often told that all the contents "ran away," and that therefore emptying was not required!

These privies are often close to the well—one within a yard of the cottagers' pump.

Earth closets are the exception, cess-pit privies the rule. [In another place 109 cess-pit privies were counted to 120 cottages. And, as might be expected, there was hardly a pure well in the place.]

In one, a market town, there *are* water-closets, so called from being without water.

Storage of Refuse and Ashes.—Ashpits are conspicuous by their absence. Huge heaps of accumulated refuse are found piled up near the house, sometimes under the windows, or near the well, into which these refuse heaps soak. Where there *are* ashpits, they are piled up and overflowing. Privy contents are often mixed up with the refuse or buried in a hole in the refuse-heap.

As to the *final disposal*, in most cases the cottagers have allotments, but differing in distance from but a few yards to as much as two miles from their homes. Their privy contents and ash refuse are therefore valuable as manure, and they would "strongly resent" any appropriation of it by the Sanitary Authority.

And we might take this into account by passing a bye-law to the effect that house refuse must be removed at least once a quarter, and that if the occupier neglected to do this, the Sanitary Authority would do it, *and would appropriate it.* This amount of pressure is thoroughly legitimate to protect the lives of the children.

Health Missioners might teach the value of co-operation in sanitary matters. For instance, suppose the hire of a sewage-cart is 1s. the first day, and sixpence every other day. If six houses, adjacent to each other, subscribed for the use of the sewage-cart, they would each get it far cheaper than by single orders.

The usual practice is to wait until there is a sufficient accumulation to make worth while the hiring of a cart. The ashes, and often the privy contents too, are then taken away to the allotments. A statement that removal takes place as much as two or three times a year is often too obviously untrue.

But, as a rule, the occupiers have sufficient garden space, *i.e.* curtilage, for the proper utilisation of their privy contents. [I would urge the reading of Dr. Poore's "Rural Hygiene" on this particular point.]

Often the garden is large enough for the utilisation of ashes and house refuse too. But occupiers almost always take both privy and ashpit contents to their allotments. Thus hoarding-up of refuse matters occurs. In some cases the cost of hiring horse and cart—the amount depending on the distance of the allotment from the dwelling—is so serious a consideration that if bye-laws compelled the occupiers to remove their refuse to their allotments, say every month, either the value of the manure would be nothing, or the scavenging must be done at the expense of the Sanitary Authority. From the public health point of view, the Sanitary Authority should of course do the scavenging in all the villages.

The health Economy of the Community demands the most profitable use of manure for the land. Now the most profitable use is that which permits of least waste, and if we could only regard economy in this matter in its true and broad sense, we should acknowledge that the Community is advantaged by the frequent removal of sewage refuse from the houses, where it is dangerous, to the land, where it is an essential. And if the Community is advantaged, the Community should pay for that advantage. The gain is a double one—safety in the matter of health—increase in the matter of food, besides the untold gain, moral as well as material, which results from the successful cultivation of land.

There are some villages without any gardens—barely room for a privy and ashpit. But even in these cases the occupiers generally have allotments.

Plenty of bye-laws may be imposed, but bye-laws are not in themselves active agents. And in many, perhaps in most, cases they are impossible of execution, and remain a dead letter.

Now let us come to

3. What the Women have to do with it—*i.e.* how much the cottage mothers, if instructed by instructed women, can remedy or prevent of these and other frightful evils.

And first

(1) Our Homes.—The Cottage Homes of England being, after all, the most important of the homes of any class, should be pure in every sense. Boys and girls must grow up healthy, with clean minds, and clean bodies, and clean skins. And the first teachings and impressions they have at home must all be pure, and gentle, and firm.

It is *home* that teaches the child after all, more than any other schooling. A child learns before it is three whether it shall obey its mother or not. And before it is seven its character is a good way to being formed.

When a child has lost its health, how often the mother says:

"O, if I had only known, but there was no one to tell me!"

God did not intend all mothers to be accompanied by doctors, but He meant all children to be cared for by mothers.

(a) *Back Yard and Garden.*—Where and how are slops emptied? The following are some of the essential requisites: slops to be poured slowly down a drain, not hastily thrown down to make a pool round the drain; gratings of drain to be kept clean and passage free; soil round the house kept pure, that pure air may come in at the window; bedroom slops not to be thrown out of window; no puddles to be allowed to stand round walls; privy contents to be got into the soil as soon as possible—most valuable for your *garden*; cesspools not to be allowed to filter into your shallow wells; pump-water wells must be taken care of, they are upright drains, so soil round them should be pure. Bad smells are danger-signals. *Pig-sties*—Moss litter to absorb liquid manure, cheap and profitable; danger from pools of liquid manure making the whole soil foul.

Now, what have we to teach practically about the

(1b) *Bedroom?*—Is not what we want to get *into* a bedroom, fresh air, the most important thing of all, and sunshine, not merely light, but sunlight? What we want to get *out of* a bedroom, foul air? An unaired bedroom is a box of foul air. Opening of windows: but windows differ so much in their construction one from the other, that no general rule can be laid down, except that in all cases there must be ventilation near the ceiling; and the Health Missioner must see the kind of window and how it opens, in order to show the best way of airing the room. If, happily, there is a fireplace, no board or sack must fill up the chimney.

Furniture of Bedroom—Bed and Bedding.—No feather or flock bed to be allowed with unwashed tick, or which has not been pulled to pieces for years to be cleaned. Cleansing of chamber utensils—danger of unemptied slops—how to get rid of dust, and not merely to let it fly into the air and settle again. How to get rid of vermin. Lumber—not to turn the space under the bed into a lumber closet with rags and refuse, worn-out clothes and boots, coals and potatoes. Nothing to be kept under the bed but the chamber utensil with a lid. No vallance, only a frill. No carpet in the bedroom. Fresh air and sunshine in the bedroom by day promote sleep by night.

(1c) *Kitchen.*—Danger from refuse of food, grease in all the rough parts of kitchen table and chopping blocks, crumbs and scraps in chinks of ill-laid floor. Even typhoid has been known to result from this in barrack-rooms. How to fill up these chinks. Danger of remains of sour milk in jugs and saucepans. All refuse poisons the air, spoils fresh food, attracts vermin, rats, beetles, &c. Brick floor too porous, dangerous to sluice with too much water. Where do you get your water for cooking? Is it water *plus* sewage? Where do you get your milk? Is it milk *plus* water *plus* sewage? Where do you keep it? How to keep milk cool; how to clean kitchen table, crockery, pots and pans. Danger of dirty sink.

Parlour.—Danger of uninhabited rooms without sunlight and fresh air, and with blinds pulled down—genteel parlour chilling to the bone. Clean papers not to be put over dirty ones. Tea-leaves for sweeping carpets; but better to have no carpets nailed down.

(2a) Ourselves.—*The Skin and How to Keep the Body Clean.*— Simple account of functions of skin. Beauty dependent on healthy state of skin, not on a fine hat. Use of the skin as throwing out waste matter. Compare the village child with a beautiful clean skin—such a child as any mother would long to kiss—with the leper of the Scriptures, a loathsome object, the skin all sores, so repulsive to others, so painful to himself, that, as a miracle, he asks to be made "*clean*," and the gracious answer comes: "I will: be thou clean."

Then show that the difference between the child and the leper is just the difference between a healthy and unhealthy skin. The difference between a clean skin and a dirty skin is the difference between health and sickness.

Enter fully but not learnedly into the work of the *pores.* Dangers of a choked skin. The body choked and poisoned by its own waste substances might be compared to a house whence nothing was thrown away—the scullery choked with old fat, potato peelings, &c., the drain from the sink stopped up, the grate full of cinders, the floor of dust, the table of grease and crumbs. None of these things were dirty at first: it is the keeping them that makes the house uninhabitable.

Then speak very plainly of the offensive condition of an unwashed body, the smell of the feet, the horrible state of the hair, the decay and pain in the teeth, &c.; the consequent poisoning of the air of the room, &c. It is the human body that pollutes the air.

Then, *how* and *when* the body can best be washed; large vessels and much water not indispensable for daily cleansing. But there are great advantages in the Saturday's tub and plenty of soaping, and in friction of the skin. Not babies only, but men and women require daily washing. The body the source of defilement of the air.

The entire want of privacy in the bedrooms, the constant drive of the mother's occupations, make it a matter of difficulty when *she* can wash herself. [As a matter of fact, most women do not wash at all.] The Missioners should show the utmost sympathy—should, without giving offence, draw her out by careful questions, asking what plan the women would *recommend* rather than what they *do*.

Then comes the question of towels.

Then comes the question of hair and hair-brushes. Mothers should encourage their girls' natural wish to look nice, make them proud of beautifully brushed and well-plaited hair, rather than of the smart hat above it.

Then comes the question of tooth-brushes. [How often does it happen that the lady's own underservants come to her service without a tooth-brush?]

The Missioner should be able to give the price of each article she recommends—towels, hair-brushes, tooth-brushes, &c.

(2*b*) *Clothes.—The Circulation, and How to Keep the Body Warm.*—Simple account of how the heart and lungs act. Clothes to be warm and loose—no pressure. Test for tight lacing: if measurement round the waist is more with the clothes off than when stays are worn. Danger of dirty clothes next the skin—re-absorption of poison; danger of wearing the same underclothing day and night; best materials for clothing—why flannel is so valuable; danger of sitting in wet clothes and boots—*too little air causes more chills than too much*; the body not easily chilled when warm and well clothed.

(2c) *Food.—The Digestion, and How to Nourish the Body.*— Simple account of how food is digested and turned into blood. Worse food (well cooked) and fresh air better than best food (ill cooked) without fresh air. Diet, not medicine, ensures health. Uses of animal and of vegetable food. Danger of all ill-cooked and half-cooked food. Nourishing value of vegetables and whole-meal bread. Danger of too little food and too much at the wrong times. Dangers of uncooked meat, specially pork, diseased meat, decaying fish, unripe and over-ripe fruit, and *stewed tea*. Vital importance of cooked fruit for children, stewed apples and pears, damsons, blackberries. *Value of milk as food.* [Don't sell all your milk.] Influence of diet upon constipation, diarrhœa, indigestion, convulsions in children; small changes of diet promote appetite and health.

(3a) Extra Subjects.—*Home Treatment.—What to do till the Doctor comes and after the Doctor has left.*—Grave danger of being one's own doctor, of taking quack medicines, or a medicine which has cured someone else in quite a different case.

A cottage mother, not so very poor, fell into the fire in a fit while she was preparing breakfast, and was badly burnt. We sent for the nearest doctor, who came at once, bringing his medicaments, in his gig. The husband ran for the horse-doctor, who did not come, but sent an ointment for a horse. The wise woman of the village came of her own accord, and gave another ointment.

"Well, Mrs. Y.," said the lady who sent for the doctor, "and what did you do?"

"Well, you know, Miss, I studied a bit, and then I mixed all three together, because then, you know, I was sure I got the right one."

The consequences to the poor woman may be imagined.

Another poor woman, in a different county, took something which had been sent to her husband for a bad leg, believing herself to have fever. "Well, Miss, it did he a sight of good, and look at me, ban't I quite peart?" The "peartness" ended in fever.

Liquid food only to be given till the doctor comes. Danger-signals of illness, and how to recognise them. Hourly dangers from ruptures if not completely supported by trusses. What to do if clothes catch fire—and for burns, scalds, bites, cuts, stings, injuries to the head and to the eye, swallowing fruit-stones, pins, &c. Simple rules to avoid infection. After the doctor has left—how to take care of convalescents; how to feed. It is not uncommon to give such things as onion broth or solid food to people and children recovering from typhoid (enteric fever), which generally produces a relapse, sometimes fatal. In convalescent homes for children the urchins have refused their bread and milk and asked for pickles (which seem now to have taken the place of sweets), and when they have found that only bread and milk was to be had for breakfast, these urchins have gone out and succeeded in getting pickles, and even kippered fish, and the like, after breakfast. When to keep rooms dark, and when to admit plenty of light. Danger of chills.

(3b) *Management of Infants and Children.*—How to feed, clothe, and wash. Nursing, weaning, hand-feeding; regular intervals between feeding; flatulence, thrush, convulsions, bronchitis, croup. Simple hints to mothers about healthy conditions for children. Baths. Diet—how to prevent constipation and diarrhœa. What to do in sudden attacks of convulsions and croup. Deadly danger of giving "soothing syrups" or alcohol. *Made* foods not wholesome. Head-ache often caused by bad eyesight. Symptoms of overwork at school—head-ache, worry, talking in the sleep. Danger to babies and little children of any violence, jerks and sudden movements, loud voices, slaps, box on the ear. Good effects upon the health of gentleness, firmness, and cheerfulness. No child can be well who is not bright and merry, and brought up in fresh air and sunshine, and surrounded by love—the sunshine of the soul.

4. (*In answer to many questions asked.*) Some Sketch of the Scheme of Health-at-Home Training and Work.—The questions asked have been mainly: How to begin? What is your plan for Health-at-Home instruction and training the Health Missioners to train the cottage mothers in their homes: it is altogether different from nursing disease: it is preventing disease. The answer must needs be somewhat dry:

(1) First and foremost the pivot must be: a rural Medical Officer of Health chosen for fitness and experience by the proper local authority.

(2) The keys to the whole situation are the educated women desirous of becoming Health Missioners, to whom lectures, training in the village itself, are given by the earnest Medical Officer of Health.

(2*a*) The lectures by the Medical Officer to include elementary physiology: *i.e.* a simple explanation of the organs of the body—how each affects the health of the body, and how each can be kept in order. This constitutes the science of Hygiene, framed so as to give the practical scientific basis on which popular familiar teaching to village mothers and girls can be given. Other ladies may be admitted to this course of not less than fifteen lectures.

(2*b*) The Medical Officer of Health gives further instruction in classes to those who wish to qualify as Health Missioners, both by oral instruction and papers.

(2*c*) The Medical Officer now takes those who have attended the classes into the villages to visit the cottages, and shows them what to observe and how to visit.

If the Medical Officer is himself in touch with the village mothers, not only will he not give offence, but these visits will be welcomed.

127

(2*d*) The Medical Officer chooses the candidates he deems qualified to be examined for Health Missioners. These qualifications must be—good character, good health, personal fitness for teaching, tact and power, so as to be "in touch" and in love with the village mothers—to be acceptable to them— growing in sympathy for them, to be their personal friend, and to make them her personal friends—not "prying about," as the village mothers might say. Not Bacteriology, but looking into the drains, is the thing needed. Even Medical Students do not learn much from lectures, unless with the objects before them. [N.B. Both Medical Officer and Missioners must be enthusiasts in the work, must believe in Hygiene and Sanitation, believe in them as a life-and-death matter.]

(3) The candidates are now examined by an independent Examiner appointed by the local authority—one who is familiar with the conditions of rural and village life, so unlike town life— who then, in conjunction with the Medical Officer, recommends the candidates who have satisfied them both to the local authority, and the latter appoints as many as are required.

(4) The Health Missioners are appointed to districts, consisting each of a number of small villages grouped with a larger one, or the market town. Over these there is a District Committee which is represented on the local authority. Each village has a local committee, represented on the District Committee. The local committee makes arrangements for the lectures by the Health Missioner and for receiving her.

(5) The Health Missioner works under the supervision of the Medical Officer of Health, who as often as possible introduces her to the village in the first instance; and he makes it his business to inquire into the practical results of her work.

(6) The lectures to the cottage mothers are delivered in simple, homely language.

But (7) the lecture is only the beginning of the work, the prelude to it. The real work is when, having made friends with the cottage mothers, and being invited by them to their own homes, every one of whom and every one of which differs from every other, the Health Missioner *practically* shows the cottage mother *there*, in the bedroom, in the kitchen and parlour, in the backyard and garden, in washing everybody's skin clean, in clothing and food—aided by the cottage mothers, who alone can tell *her* how to make what she has taught *practicable*. They teach her as much as she teaches them. The mothers should help her by asking questions and by relating their own experiences. And, in a lecture, the Missioner should welcome such questions, even if asked rudely. If she snubs them, it is all over with her usefulness.

The eye and hand must be trained to see and deal with dangers to health. "No practical knowledge is possible on any subject without the meeting of the senses with the material."

(8) After a Health Missioner has become settled in a district, she will then be able to receive a Probationer, who, while attending the Medical Officer's lectures and classes, will find time to accompany the Health Missioner in her round of visiting. [It will depend on the tact of the two ladies if this is acceptable or not to the cottage mother; if unacceptable, it must, of course, cease.] The Lecturing Missioner must be well acquainted with the busy life of cottage mothers. The contrast is indeed strange between the poor woman who said (she was every day thirteen to fifteen hours on her feet), "O that I could sit down one hour a day, with nothing to do!" and the young lady who has her arms and legs pulled about by "Kinesipathy," or some such conundrum, to supply the want of exercise.

(9) You will doubtless ask: How shall we get the results of the Health Missioner's work fairly and completely tested? A question not at all easy to answer, because, in the first place, there can be no speedy results, the process is necessarily very slow; and because, in the second place, the results are often not on the surface, but in the intimate and private habits of life which a stranger who comes on a tour of inspection can hardly inquire about without giving offence. There are, however, two kinds of tests. The one is that which a carefully prepared system of written

returns will give, showing attendance at village lectures, and the number of cottage visits paid by invitation, and other figures and facts that are capable of tabulation. The other test is that which can be obtained from a tactful Lady Visitor, who may go round either with (if she be a stranger to the people) or on the track of the Health Missioner, gathering as she goes, by the talk of those whom she visits and the condition of their cottages, what the influence of the Health Missioner has been, and how she has bettered the facts and conditions of the lives of the people.

5. What we Mean by Personal Acquaintance and Friendship between the Lady Lecturers and Cottage Mothers.—This is not to be made by lecturing upon bedrooms, sculleries, sties, and wells *in general*; but by actual examination of the particular bedroom, scullery, sty, and well, which differ as much in different cottages as the characters of the inmates. A lecturer is a prescribing person. But what would you say of a prescribing doctor who only saw his or her patient on the benches of a room, who never examined into the case of each individual, never visited his patients, or came into touch with any of them? This is the lecturer. He or she is not even a tutor who sees pupils separately. He or she never comes into contact with them. To the lectured mother it is like going to the play. The cottage mother is, as a rule, both civil and timid. But how often one has heard her say: "I be sure it's very kind of the ladies to come and lecture to we, or try to amuse we. But that's not what we want. *They* don't know what us wants." Sympathy with, interest in the poor so as to help them, can only be got by long and close intercourse with each in her own house—not patronising—not "talking down" to them—not "prying about;" sympathy which will grow in insight and love with every visit; which will enable you to *show* the cottage mother on the spot how to give air to the bedroom, &c. *You* could not get through the daily work of the cottage mother—the washing, cooking, cleaning, mending, making. So ask what plan *she* would *recommend* to carry out your suggestions rather than what she *does*. The old cottage mother has no idea

of responsibility for the health of her family. It is all the "will of God." But the young mother, who has had some education, is anxious to be taught. A very pregnant remark was made: "How superior the animal mother is to the human mother in intelligent care of her offspring; the cow never tries to teach her calf to eat grass, and the cat licks her kitten all over before it is half-an-hour old." As has been said of other people, may yet more truly be said of cottage mothers. You cannot know them by just seeing them in class. You certainly cannot know their homes, their circumstances, their daily work so excessive, their troubles so bravely borne, their gossip—often their only recreation. *You cannot know the points through which they can be influenced and influence others.* They certainly cannot be managed or influenced in a lump—rather less than anybody else. You must know each and her individuality, separately at home, if you are to do any good. And you must be welcome to them. You must "mother" the cottage mothers, and the girls. And don't think that the gain is all on their side. How much we learn from the poor—how much from our patients in hospital—when heart meets heart. It is a rule among the best District Nurse Societies not to give alms (money). This also should be a rule of the Health Missioners. But without knowing the wants, the difficulties, temptations, fatigues, of their daily lives—without a serious study of their world—we cannot help them. Much fatigue is occasioned by their want of method. Their deplorable manners to their children have been noticed. "I'll bray your brains out if you don't do it *voluntally*"— this was an affectionate mother, about going to school. But then, the heroism of the poor! The lecture is only a foothold for knowing the cottage mothers. And let us remember the town can no more instruct the country than the country the town. The success of this or any work cannot be tested by the number of lectures delivered, or even by the attendance at the lectures, but only by the practical results that have actually appeared from the teaching *applied* in personal visits. Such results must of course be slow; but slow and sure wins the race. The test of success is the gaining the confidence of the village mothers, and being invited to help them in their own homes. They must feel that the Health Missioner comes not to find fault, but to find friends. And the lectures will indeed be a dismal failure unless the cottage women support the Missioners. "It seems to be of no use talking," said a great Sanitary Commissioner. And it is perfectly vain to try to convert the villagers without *themselves*. *Results shown* are the only test.

CONCLUSION.

The criticism on all this will be: "What an enormous time it will take! You are describing a process that will not take weeks, but months and years. Life is not long enough for this."

Our reply is that, for centuries there have been superstitions, for centuries the habits of dirt and neglect have been steadily and perseveringly learnt, and that, if we can transform by a few years' quiet persistent work the habits of centuries, the process will not have been slow, but amazingly rapid. What is "slow" in more senses than one is the eternal lecturing that is *vox et præterea nihil*—words that go in at one ear and out at the other. The only word that sticks is the word that follows work. The work that "pays" is the work of the skilful hand, directed by the cool head, and inspired by the loving heart. Join heart with heart and hand in hand, and pray for the perfect gift of love to be the spirit and the life of all your work.

Can there be any higher work than this? Can any woman wish for a more womanly work? Can any man think it unworthy of the best of women?

When the greatest men of science devote a large part of their lives to bring in simple language within the reach of all the results of their deepest study, the women of the highest cultivation and of the deepest sympathy may well take up such work as we have attempted here to sketch out.

But they must "stoop to conquer." Or rather, they must not think it "stooping," but following the Divine in their hearts, to be "at home" in the cottage mothers' homes.

FLORENCE NIGHTINGALE TO HER NURSES

I

London, May, 1872.

For us who Nurse, our Nursing is a thing, which, unless in it we are making *progress* every year, every month, every week, take my word for it we are going *back*.

The more experience we gain, the more progress we can make. The progress you make in your year's training with us is as nothing to what you must make every year *after* your year's training is over.

A woman who thinks in herself: "Now I am a 'full' Nurse, a 'skilled' Nurse, I have learnt all that there is to be learnt": take my word for it, she does not know *what a Nurse is*, and she never *will* know; she is *gone* back already.

Conceit and Nursing cannot exist in the same person, any more than new patches on an old garment.

Every year of her service a good Nurse will say: "I learn something every day."

I have had more experience in all countries and in different ways of Hospitals than almost any one ever had before (there were no opportunities for learning in *my* youth such as you have had); but if I could recover strength so much as to walk about, I would begin all over again. I would come for a year's training to St. Thomas' Hospital under your admirable Matron (and I

134

venture to add that she would find me the closest in obedience to all our rules), sure that I should learn every day, learn all the more for my past experience.

And then I would try to be learning every day to the last hour of my life. "And when his legs were cuttit off, He fought upon his stumps," says the ballad; so, when I could no longer learn by nursing others, I would learn by being nursed, by seeing Nurses practise upon *me*. It is all experience.

Agnes Jones, who died as Matron of the Liverpool Workhouse Infirmary (whom you may have heard of as "Una"), wrote from the Workhouse in the last year of her life: "I mean to stay at this post forty years, God willing; but I must come back to St. Thomas' as soon as I have a holiday; I shall learn so much more" (she had been a year at St. Thomas') "now that I have more experience."

When I was a child, I remember reading that Sir Isaac Newton, who was, as you know, perhaps the greatest discoverer among the Stars and the Earth's wonders who ever lived, said in his last hours: "I seem to myself like a child who has been playing with a few pebbles on the sea-shore, leaving unsearched all the wonders of the great Ocean beyond."

By the side of this put a Nurse leaving her Training School and reckoning up what she has learnt, ending with—"The only wonder is that one head can contain it all." (What a small head it must be then!)

I seem to have remembered all through life Sir Isaac Newton's words.

And to nurse—that is, under Doctor's orders, to cure or to prevent sickness and maiming, Surgical and Medical,—is a field, a road, of which one may safely say: There is no end-no end in what we may be learning every day.[2]

I have sometimes heard: "But have we not reason to be conceited, when we compare ourselves to ... and ...?" (naming drinking, immoral, careless, dishonest Nurses). I will not think it possible that such things can ever be said among *us*.

Taking it even upon the worldly ground, what woman among us, instead of looking to that which is higher, will of her own accord compare herself with that which is lower—with immoral women?

Does not the Apostle say: "I count not myself to have apprehended: but this one thing I do, forgetting those things which are behind, *and reaching forth unto those things which are before, I press toward* the mark for the prize of the *high calling* of God in Christ Jesus"; and what higher "calling" can we have than Nursing? But then we must "press forward"; we have indeed *not* "apprehended" if we have not "apprehended" even so much as this.

There is a little story about "the Pharisee" known over all Christendom. Should Christ come again upon the earth, would He have to apply that parable to us?

And now, let me say a thing which I am sure must have been in all your minds before this: if, unless we improve every day in our Nursing, we are going back: how much more must it be, that, unless we improve every day in our conduct as Christian women, followers of Him by whose name we call ourselves, we shall be going back?

This applies of course to every woman in the world; but it applies more especially to us, because we know no one calling in the world, except it be that of teaching, in which *what we can do* depends so much upon *what we are.* To be *a good Nurse* one must be *a good woman;* or one is truly nothing but a tinkling bell. To be a good woman at all, one must be an improving woman; for stagnant waters sooner or later, and stagnant air, as we know ourselves, always grow corrupt and unfit for use.

Is any one of us a *stagnant woman*? Let it not have to be said by any one of us: I left this Home a worse woman than I came into it. I came in with earnest purpose, and now I think of little but my own satisfaction and a good place.

When the head and the hands are very full, as in Nursing, it is so easy, so very easy, if the heart has not an earnest purpose for God and our neighbour, to end in doing one's work only for oneself, and not at all—even when we seem to be serving our neighbours—not at all for them or for God.

I should hardly like to talk of a subject which, after all, must be very much between each one of us and her God,—which is hardly a matter for *talk* at all, and certainly not for me, who cannot be among you (though there is nothing in the world I should so dearly wish), but that I thought perhaps you might like to hear of things which persons in the same situation, that is, in different Training Schools on the Continent, have said to me.

I will mention two or three:

1. One said, "The greatest help I ever had in life was that we were taught in our Training School always to raise our hearts to God the first thing on waking in the morning."

Now it need hardly be said that we cannot make a rule for this; a rule will not teach this, any more than making a rule that the chimney shall not smoke will make the smoke go up the chimney.

If we occupy ourselves the last thing at night with rushing about, gossiping in one another's rooms; if our last thoughts at night are of some slight against ourselves, or spite against another, or about each other's tempers, it is needless to say that our first thoughts in the morning will not be of God.

Perhaps there may even have been some quarrel; and if those who pretend to be educated women indulge in these irreligious uneducated disputes, what a scandal before those less educated, to whom an example, not a stone of offence, should be set!

"A thousand irreligious cursed hours" (as some poet says), have not seldom, in the lives of all but a few whom we may truly call Saints upon earth, been spent on some feeling of ill-will. And can we expect to be really able to lift up our hearts the first thing in the morning to the God of "good will towards men" if we do this?

I speak for myself, even more perhaps than for others.

2. Another woman[3] once said to me:—"I was taught in my

Training School never to have those long inward discussions with myself, those interminable conversations inside myself, which make up so much more of our own thoughts than we are aware. If it was something about my duties, I went straight to my Superiors, and asked for leave or advice; if it was any of those useless or ill-tempered thoughts about one another, or those that were put over us, we were taught to lay them before God and get the better of them, before they got the better of us."

A spark can be put out while it is a spark, if it falls on our dress, but not when it has set the whole dress in flames. So it is with an ill-tempered thought against another. And who will tell how much of our thoughts these occupy?

I suppose, of course, that those who think themselves better than others are bent upon setting them a better example.

And this brings me to something else. (I can always correct others though I cannot always correct myself.) It is about jealousies and punctilios as to ranks, classes, and offices, when employed in one good work. What an injury this jealous woman is doing, not to others, or not to others so much as to herself; she is doing it to herself! She is not getting out of her work the advantage, the improvement to her own character, the nobleness (for to be useful is the only true nobleness) which God has appointed her that work to attain. She is not getting out of her work what God has given it her for; but just the contrary.

(Nurses are not children, but women; and if they can't do this for themselves, no one can for them.)

I think it is one of Shakespeare's heroes who says "I laboured to be wretched." How true that is! How true it is of some people all their lives; and perhaps there is not one of us who could not say it with truth of herself at one time or other: I laboured to be mean and contemptible and small and ill-tempered, by being revengeful of petty slights.

A woman once said: "What signifies it to me that this one does me an injury or the other speaks ill of me, if I do not deserve it? The injury strikes God before it strikes me, and if He forgives it, why should not I? I hope I love Him better than I do myself." This may sound fanciful; but is there not truth in it?

What a privilege it is, the work that God has given us Nurses to do, if we will only let Him have His own way with us—a greater privilege to my mind than He has given to any woman (except to those who are teachers), because *we* can always be useful, always "ministering" to others, real followers of Him who said that He came "not to be ministered unto" but to minister. Cannot we fancy Him saying to *us*, If any one thinks herself greater among you, let her minister unto others.

This is not to say that we are to be doing other people's work. Quite the reverse. The very essence of all good organisation is that everybody should do her (or his) own work in such a way as to help and not to hinder every one else's work.

But this being arranged, that any one should say, I am "put upon" by having to associate with so-and-so; or by *not* having so-and-so to associate with; or, by not having such a post; or, by having such a post; or, by my Superiors "walking upon me," or, "dancing" upon me (you may laugh, but such things have actually been said), or etc., etc.,—this is simply making the peace of God impossible, the call of God (for in all work He calls us) of none effect; it is grieving the Spirit of God; it is doing our best to make all free-will associations intolerable.

In "Religious Orders" this is provided against by enforcing blind, unconditional obedience through the fears and promises of a Church.

Does it not seem to you that the greater freedom of secular Nursing Institutions, as it requires (or ought to require) greater individual responsibility, greater self-command in each one, greater nobleness in each, greater *self-possession* in *patience*—so, that very need of self-possession, of greater nobleness in each, requires (or ought to require) greater thought in each, more discretion, and higher, not less, obedience? For the obedience of intelligence, not the obedience of slavery, is what *we* want.

The slave obeys with stupid obedience, with deceitful evasion of service, or with careless eye service. Now, we cannot suppose God to be satisfied or pleased with stupidity and carelessness. The free woman in Christ obeys, or rather *seconds* all the rules, all the orders given her, with intelligence, with all her heart, and with all her strength, and with all her *mind*.

"Not slothful in business; fervent in spirit, serving the Lord."

And you who have to be Head Nurses, or Sisters of Wards, well know what I mean, for you have to be Ward *Mistresses* as well as Nurses; and how can she (the Ward Mistress) command if she has not learnt how to obey? If she cannot enforce upon herself to obey rules with discretion, how can she enforce upon her Ward to obey rules with discretion?

And of those who have to be Ward Mistresses, as well as those who are Ward Mistresses already, or in any charge of trust or authority, I will ask, if Sisters and Head Nurses will allow me to ask of them, as I have so often asked of myself—

What is it that made our Lord speak "as one having authority"? What was the key to *His* "authority"? Is it anything which we, trying to be "like Him," could have—like Him?

What are the qualities which give us authority, which enable us to exercise some charge or control over others with "authority"? It is not the charge or position itself, for we often see persons in a position of authority, who have no authority at all; and on the other hand we sometimes see persons in the very humblest position who exercise a great influence or authority on all around them.

The very first element for having control over others is, of course, to have control over oneself. If I cannot take charge of myself, I cannot take charge of others. The next, perhaps, is—not to try to "seem" anything, but to *be* what we would *seem*.

A person in charge must be felt more than she is heard—not heard more than she is felt. She must fulfil her charge without noisy disputes, by the silent power of a consistent life, in which there is no *seeming*, and no hiding, but plenty of discretion. She must exercise authority without appearing to exercise it.

A person, but more especially a woman, in charge must have a quieter and more impartial mind than those under her, in order to influence them by the best part of them and not by the worst.

We (Sisters) think that we must often make allowances for them, and sometimes put ourselves in their place. And I will appeal to Sisters to say whether we must not observe more than we speak, instead of speaking more than we observe. We must not give an order, much less a reproof, without being fully acquainted with both sides of the case. Else, having scolded wrongfully, we look rather foolish.

The person in charge every one must see to be just and candid, looking at both sides, not moved by entreaties or, by likes and dislikes, but only by justice; and always reasonable, remembering and not forgetting the wants of those of whom she is in charge.

She must have a keen though generous insight into the characters of those she has to control. They must know that she *cares for* them even while she is checking them; or rather that she checks them *because* she cares for them. A woman *thus* reproved is often made your friend for life; a word dropped in this way by a Sister in charge (I am speaking now solely to Sisters and Head Nurses) may sometimes show a probationer the unspeakable importance of this year of her life, when she must sow the seed of her future nursing in this world, and of her future life through eternity. For although future years are of importance to train the plant and make it come up, yet if there is no seed nothing will come up.

Nay, I appeal again to Sisters' own experience, whether they have not known patients feel the same of words dropped before *them.*

We had in one of the Hospitals which we nurse a little girl patient of seven years old, the child of a bad mother, who used to pray on her knees (when she did not know she was heard) her own little prayer that she might not forget, when she went away to what she already knew to be a bad life, the good words she had been taught. (In this great London, the time that children spend in Hospital is sometimes the only time in their lives that they hear good words.) And sometimes we have had patients, widows of journeymen for instance, who had striven to the last to do for their children and place them all out in service or at work, die in our Hospitals, thanking God that they had had this time to collect their thoughts before death, and to die "so comfortably" as they expressed it.

But, if a Ward is not kept in such a spirit that patients can collect their thoughts, whether it is for life or for death, and that children can hear good words, of course these things will not happen.

Ward management is only made possible by kindness and sympathy. And the mere way in which a thing is said or done to patient, or probationer, makes all the difference. In a Ward, too, where there is no *order* there can be no "authority"; there must be noise and dispute.

Hospital Sisters are the only women who may be in charge really of men. Is this not enough to show how essential to them are those qualities which alone constitute real authority?

Never to have a quarrel with another; never to say things which rankle in another's mind; never when we are uncomfortable ourselves to make others uncomfortable—for quarrels come out of such very small matters, a hasty word, a sharp joke, a harsh order: without regard to these things, how can we take charge?

We may say, so-and-so is too weak if she minds that. But, pray, are we not weak in the same way ourselves?

I have been in positions of authority myself and have always tried to remember that to use such an advantage inconsiderately is—cowardly. To be sharp upon them is worse in me than in them to be sharp upon me. No one can trample upon others, and govern them. To win them is half, I might say the whole, secret of "having charge." If you find your way to their hearts, you may do what you like with them; and that authority is the most complete which is least perceived or asserted.

The world, whether of a Ward or of an Empire, is governed

not by many words but by few; though some, especially women, seem to expect to govern by many words—by talk, and nothing else.

There is scarcely anything which interferes so much with charge over others as rash and inconsiderate talking, or as wearing one's thoughts on one's cap. There is scarcely anything which interferes so much with their respect for us as any want of simplicity in us. A person who is always thinking of herself— how she looks, what effect she produces upon others, what others will think or say of her—can scarcely ever hope to have charge of them to any purpose.

We ought to be what we want to seem, or those under us will find out very soon that we only seem what we ought to be.

If we think only of the duty we have in hand, we may hope to make the others think of it too. But if we are fidgety or uneasy about trifles, can we hope to impress them with the importance of essential things?

There is so much talk about persons now-a-days. Everybody criticises everybody. Everybody seems liable to be drawn into a current, against somebody, or in favour of every one doing what she likes, pleasing herself, or getting promotion.

If any one gives way to all these distractions, and has no root of calmness in herself, she will not find it in any Hospital or Home.

"All this is as old as the hills," you will say. Yes, it is as old as Christianity; and is not that the more reason for us to begin to practise it to-day? "*To-day*, if ye will hear my voice," says the Father; "*To-day* ye shall be with me in Paradise," says the Son; and He does not say this only to the dying; for Heaven may begin here, and "The kingdom of heaven is within," He tells us.

Most of you here present will be in a few years in charge of others, filling posts of responsibility. *All* are on the threshold of active life. Then our characters will be put to the test, whether in some position of charge or of subordination, or both. Shall we be found wanting? Unable to control ourselves, therefore unable to control others? With many good qualities, perhaps, but owing to selfishness, conceit, to some want of purpose, some laxness, carelessness, lightness, vanity, some temper, habits of self-indulgence, or want of disinterestedness, unequal to the struggle of life, the business of life, and ill-adapted to the employment of Nursing, which we have chosen for ourselves, and which, almost above all others, requires earnest purpose, and the reverse of all these faults? Thirty years hence, if we could suppose us all standing here again passing judgment on ourselves, and telling sincerely why one has succeeded and another has failed; why the life of one has been a blessing to those she has charge of, and another has gone from one thing to another, pleasing herself, and bringing nothing to good—what would we give to be able *now* to see all this before us?

Yet some of those reasons for failure or success we may anticipate now. Because so-and-so was or was not weak or vain; because she could or could not make herself respected; because she had no steadfastness in her, or on the contrary because she had a fixed and steady purpose; because she was selfish or unselfish, disliked or beloved; because she could or could not keep her women together or manage her patients, or was or was not to be trusted in Ward business. And there are many other reasons which I might give you, or which you might give yourselves, for the success or failure of those who have passed through this Training School for the last eleven years.

Can we not see ourselves as others see us?

For the "world is a hard schoolmaster," and punishes us without giving reasons, and much more severely than any Training School can, and when we can no longer perhaps correct the defect.

Good posts may be found for us; but can we keep them so as to fill them worthily? Or are we but unprofitable servants in fulfilling any charge?

Yet many of us are blinded to the truth by our own self-love even to the end. And we attribute to accident or ill-luck what is really the consequence of some weakness or error in ourselves.

But "can we not see ourselves as God sees us?" is a still more important question. For while we value the judgments of our superiors, and of our fellows, which may correct our own judgments, we must also have a higher standard which may correct theirs. We cannot altogether trust them, and still less can we trust ourselves. And we know, of course, that the worth of a life is not altogether measured by failure or success. We want to see our purposes, and the ways we take to fulfil such charge as may be given us, as they are in the sight of God. "Thou God seest me."

And thus do we return to the question we asked before— how near can we come to Him whose name we bear, when we call ourselves Christians? How near to His gentleness and goodness—to His "authority" over others.[4]

And the highest "authority" which a woman especially can attain among her fellow women must come from her doing God's work here in the same spirit, and with the same thoroughness, that Christ did, though we follow him but "afar off."

Lastly, it is charity to nurse sick bodies well; it is greater charity to nurse well and patiently sick minds, tiresome sufferers. But there is a greater charity even than these: to do good to those who are not good to us, to behave well to those who behave ill to us, to serve with love those who do not even receive our service with good temper, to forgive on the instant any slight which we may have received, or may have fancied we have received, or any worse injury.

If we cannot "do good" to those who "persecute" us—for we are not "persecuted": if we cannot pray "Father, forgive them, for they know not what they do"—for none are nailing us to a cross: how much more must we try to serve with patience and love any who use us spitefully, to nurse with all our hearts any thankless peevish patients!

We Nurses may well call ourselves "blessed among women" in this, that we can be always exercising all these three charities, and so fulfil the work our God has given us to do.

Just as I was writing this came a letter from Mrs. Beecher Stowe, who wrote *Uncle Tom's Cabin*. She has so fallen in love with the character of our Agnes Jones ("Una")[5] which she had just read, that she asks about the progress of our work, supposing that we have many more Unas. They wish to "organise a similar movement" in America—a "movement" of Unas—what a great thing that would be! Shall we all try to be Unas?

She ends, as I wish to end,—"Yours, in the dear name that is above every other,"

FLORENCE NIGHTINGALE.

II

May 23, 1873.

My dear Friends,—Another year has passed over us. Nearly though not quite all of us who were here at this time last year have gone their several ways, to their several posts; some at St. Thomas', some to Edinburgh, some to Highgate. Nearly all are, I am thankful to say, well, and I hope we may say happy. Some are gone altogether.

May this year have set us all one step farther, one year on our way to becoming "perfect as our Father in Heaven is perfect," as it ought to have done.

Some differences have been made in the School by our good Matron, who toils for us early and late—to bring us on the way, we hope, towards becoming "perfect."

These differences—I leave it to you to say, improvements—are as you see: our new Medical Instructor having vigorously taken us in hand and giving us his invaluable teaching (1) in Medical and Surgical Nursing, (2) in the elements of Anatomy. I need not say: Let us profit.

Next, in order to give more time and leisure to less tired bodies, the Special Probationers have two afternoons in the week off duty for the course of reading which our able Medical Instructor has laid down. And the Nurse-Probationers have all one morning and one afternoon in the week to improve themselves, in which our kind Home Sister assists them by classes. And, again, I need not say how important it is to take the utmost advantage of this. Do not let the world move on and leave us in the wrong. Now that, by the law of the land, every child between five and thirteen must be at school, it will be a poor tale, indeed, in their after life for Nurses who cannot read, write, spell, and cypher well and correctly, and read aloud easily, and take notes of the temperature of cases, and the like. Only this last week, I was told by one of our own Matrons of an excellent Nurse of her own to whom she would have given a good place, only that she could neither read nor write well enough for it.

And may I tell you, not for envy, but for a generous rivalry, that you will have to work hard if you wish St. Thomas' Training School to hold its own with other Schools rising up.

Let us be on our guard against the danger, not exactly of thinking too well of ourselves (for no one consciously does this), but of isolating ourselves, of falling into party spirit—always remembering that, if we can do any good to others, we must draw others to us by the influence of our characters, and not by any profession of what we are—least of all, by a profession of Religion.

And this, by the way, applies peculiarly to what we are with our patients. Least of all should a *woman* try to exercise religious influence with her patients, as it were, by a ministry, a chaplaincy. We are not chaplains. It is what she *is* in *herself*, and what comes out of herself, out of what she *is*—that exercise a moral or religious influence over her patients. No set form of words is of any use. And patients are so quick to see whether a Nurse is consistent always in herself—whether she *is* what she *says* to them. And if she is not, it is no use. *If she is*, of how much use, unawares to herself, may the simplest word of soothing, of comfort, or even of reproof—especially in the quiet night—be to the roughest patient, who is there from drink, or to the still innocent child, or to the anxious toil-worn mother or husband! But if she wishes to do this, she must keep up a sort of divine calm and high sense of duty in her own mind. Christ was alone, from time to time, in the wilderness or on mountains. If *He* needed this, how much more must we?

Quiet in our own rooms (and a room of your own is specially provided for each one here); a few minutes of calm thought to offer up the day to God: how indispensable it is, in this ever increasing hurry of life! When we live "so fast," do we not require a breathing time, a moment or two daily, to think where we are going? At this time, especially, when we are laying the foundation of our after life, in reality the most important time of all.

And I am not at all saying that our patients have everything to learn from *us*. On the contrary, we can, many a time, learn from them, in patience, in true religious feeling and hope. One of our Sisters told me that she had often learnt more from her patients than from any one else. And I am sure I can say the same for myself. The poorest, the meanest, the humblest patient may enter into the kingdom of Heaven before the cleverest of us, or the most conceited. For, in another world, many, many of the conditions of this world must be changed. Do we think of this?

We have been, almost all of us, taught to pray in the days of our childhood. Is there not something sad and strange in our throwing this aside when most required by us, on the threshold of our active lives? Life is a shallow thing, and more especially *Hospital* life, without any depth of religion. For it is a matter of simple experience that the best things, the things which seem as if they most would make us feel, become the most hardening if not rightly used.

And may I say a thing from my own experience? No training is of any use, unless one can learn (1) to feel, and (2) to think out things for oneself. And if we have not true religious feeling and purpose, Hospital life—the highest of all things *with* these—*without* them becomes a mere routine and bustle, and a very hardening routine and bustle.

One of our past Probationers said: "Our work must be the first thing, but God must be in it." "And He is not in it," she added. But let us hope that this is not so. I am sure it was not so with *her*. Let us try to make it not so with any of us.

There are three things which one must have to prevent this degeneration in oneself. And let each one of us, from time to time, tell, not any one else, but herself, whether she has these less or more than when she began her training here.

One is the real, deep, religious feeling and strong, personal, motherly interest for each one of our patients. And you can see this motherly interest in girls of twenty-one—we have had Sisters of not more than that age who had it—and *not* see it in women of forty.

The second is a strong practical (intellectual, if you will) interest in the *case*, how it is going on. This is what makes the true Nurse. Otherwise the patients might as well be pieces of furniture, and we the housemaids, unless we see how interesting a thing Nursing is. This is what makes us urge you to begin to observe the very first case you see.

The third is the pleasures of administration, which, though a fine word, means only learning to manage a Ward well: to keep it fresh, clean, tidy; to keep up its good order, punctuality; to report your cases with absolute accuracy to the Surgeon or Physician, and first to report them to the Sister; and to do all that is contained in the one word, Ward-management: to keep wine-lists, diet-lists, washing-lists—that is Sister's work—and to do all the things no less important which constitute Nurse's work.

But it would take a whole book for me to count up these; and I am going back to the first thing that we were saying: without deep religious purpose how shallow a thing is Hospital life, which is, or ought to be, the most inspiring! For, as years go on, we shall have others to train; and find that the springs of religion are dried up within ourselves. The patients we shall always have with us while we are Nurses. And we shall find that we have no religious gift or influence with them, no word in season, whether for those who are to live, or for those who are to die, no, not even when they are in their last hours, and perhaps no one by but *us* to speak a word to point them to the Eternal Father and Saviour; not even for a poor little dying child who cries: "Nursey, tell me, oh, why is it so dark?" Then we may feel painfully about them what we do not at present feel about ourselves. We may wish, both for our patients and Probationers, that they had the restraints of the "fear" of the most Holy God, to enable them to resist the temptation. We may regret that our own Probationers seem so worldly and external. And we may perceive too late that the deficiency in their characters began in our own.

For, to all good women, *life* is a prayer; and though we pray in our own rooms, in the Wards and at Church, the end must not be confounded with the means. We are the more bound to watch strictly over ourselves; we have not less but more need of a high standard of duty and of life in our Nursing; we must teach ourselves humility and modesty by becoming more aware of our own weakness and narrowness, and liability to mistake as Nurses and as Christians. Mere worldly success to any nobler, higher mind is not worth having. Do you think Agnes Jones, or some who are now living amongst us, cared much about worldly success? They cared about efficiency, thoroughness. But that is a different thing.

We must condemn many of our own tempers when we calmly review them. We must lament over training opportunities which we have lost, must desire to become better women, better Nurses. That we all of us must feel. And then, and not till then, will *life* and *work* among the sick become a prayer.

For prayer is communion or co-operation with God: the expression of a *life* among his poor and sick and erring ones. But when we speak with God, our power of addressing Him, of holding communion with Him, and listening to His still small voice, depends upon our will being one and the same with His. *Is* He our God, as He was Christ's? To Christ He was all, to us He seems sometimes nothing. Can we retire to rest after our busy, anxious day in the Wards, with the feeling: "Lord, into Thy hands I commend my spirit," and those of such and such anxious cases; remembering, too, that in the darkness, "Thou God seest me," and seest them too? Can we rise in the morning, almost with a feeling of joy that we are spared another day to do Him service with His sick?—

> Awake, my soul, and with the sun,
> Thy daily stage of duty run.

Does the thought ever occur to us in the course of the day, that we will correct that particular fault of mind, or heart, or temper, whether slowness, or bustle, or want of accuracy or method, or harsh judgments, or want of loyalty to those under whom or among whom we are placed, or sharp talking, or tale-bearing or gossiping—oh, how common, and how old a fault, as old as Solomon! "He that repeateth a matter, separateth friends;" and how can people trust us unless they know that we are not tale-bearers, who will misrepresent or improperly repeat what is said to us? Shall we correct this, or any other fault, not with a view to our success in life, or to our own credit, but in order that we may be able to serve our Master better in the service of the sick? Or do we ever seek to carry on the battle against light behaviour, against self-indulgence, against evil tempers (the "world," the "flesh," and the "devil"), and the temptations that beset us; conscious that in ourselves we are weak, but that there is a strength greater than our own, "which is perfected in weakness"? Do we think of God as the Eternal, into whose hands our patients, whom we see dying in the Wards, must resign their souls—into whose hands we must resign our own when we depart hence, and ought to resign our own as entirely every morning and night of our lives here; with whom do live the spirits of the just made perfect, with whom do really live, *ought* really as much to live, our spirits here, and who, in the hour of death, in the hour of life, both for our patients and ourselves, must be our trust and hope? We would not always be thinking of death, for "we must live before we die," and life, perhaps, is as difficult as death. Yet the thought of a time when we shall have passed out of the sight and memory of men may also help us to live; may assist us in shaking off the load of tempers, jealousies, prejudices, bitternesses, interests which weigh us down; may teach us to rise out of this busy, bustling Hospital world, into the clearer light of God's Kingdom, of which, indeed, this Home is or might be a part, and certainly and especially this Hospital.

This is the spirit of prayer, the spirit of conversation or communion with God, which leads us in all our Nursing silently to think of Him, and refer it to Him. When we hear in the voice of conscience *His* voice speaking to us; when we are aware that He is the witness of everything we do, and say, and think, and also the source of every good thing in us; and when we feel in our hearts the struggle against some evil temper, then God is fighting *with* us against envy and jealousy, against selfishness and self-indulgence, against lightness, and frivolity, and vanity, for "our better self against our worse self."

And thus, too, the friendships which have begun at this School may last through life, and be a help and strength to us. For may we not regard the opportunity given for acquiring friends as one of the uses of this place? and Christian friendship, in uniting us to a friend, as uniting us at the same time to Christ and God? Christ called His disciples friends, adding the reason, "because He had told them all that He had heard of the Father," just as women tell their whole mind to their friends.

But we all know that there are dangers and disappointments in friendships, especially in women's friendships, as well as joys and sorrows. A woman may have an honourable desire to know those who are her superiors in education, in the School, or in

Nursing. Or she may allow herself to drop into the society of those beneath her, perhaps because she is more at home with them, and is proud or shy with her superiors. We do not want to be judges of our fellow-women (for who made thee to differ from another?), but neither can we leave entirely to chance one of the greatest interests of human life.

True friendship is simple, womanly, unreserved: not weak, or silly, or fond, or noisy, or romping, or extravagant, nor yet jealous and selfish, and exacting more than woman's nature can fairly give, for there are other ties which bind women to one another besides friendship; nor, again, intrusive into the secrets of another woman, or curious about her circumstances; rejoicing in the presence of a friend, and not forgetting her in her absence.

Two Probationers or Nurses going together have not only a twofold, but a fourfold strength, if they learn knowledge or good from one another; if they form the characters of one another; if they support one another in fulfilling the duties and bearing the troubles of a Nursing life, if their friendship thus becomes fellow-service to God in their daily work. They may sometimes rejoice together over the portion of their training which has been accomplished, and take counsel about what remains to be done. They will desire to keep one another up to the mark; not to allow idleness or eccentricity to spoil their time of training.

But some of our youthful friendships are too violent to last: they have in them something of weakness or sentimentalism; the feeling passes away, and we become ashamed of them. Or at some critical time a friend has failed to stand by us, and then it is useless to talk of "auld lang syne." Only still let us remember that there are duties which we owe to the "extinct" friend (who perhaps on some fanciful ground has parted company from us), that we should never speak against her, or make use of our knowledge about her. For the memory of a friendship is like the memory of a dead friend, not lightly to be spoken of.

And then there is the "Christian or ideal friendship." What others regard as the service of the sick she may recognise as also the service of God; what others do out of compassion for their maimed fellow-creatures she may do also for the love of Christ. Feeling that God has made her what she is, she may seek to carry on her work in the Hospital as a fellow-worker with God. Remembering that Christ died for her, she may be ready to lay down her life for her patients.

"They walked together in the house of God as friends"—that is, they served God together in doing good to His sick. For if ever a place may be called the "house of God," it is a Hospital, if it be what it should be. And in old times it *was* called the "house" or the "hotel" of God. The greatest and oldest Central Hospital of Paris, where is the Mother-house of the principal Order of Nursing Sisters, is to this day called the Hôtel Dieu, the "House of God."

There may be some amongst us who, like St. Paul, are capable of feeling a natural interest in the spiritual welfare of our fellow-probationers—or, if you like the expression better, in the improvement of their characters—that they may become more such as God intended them to be in this Hospital and Home. For "Christian friendship is not merely the friendship of equals, but of unequals"—the love of the weak and of those who can make no return, like the love of God towards the unthankful and the evil. It is not a friendship of one or two but of many. It proceeds upon a different rule: "Love your enemies." It is founded upon that charity "which is not easily offended, which beareth all things, believeth all things, hopeth all things, endureth all things." Such a friendship we may be hardly able to reconcile either with our own character or with common prudence. Yet this is the "Christian ideal in the Gospel." And here and there may be found some one who has been inspired to carry out the ideal in practice.

"To live in isolation is to be weak and unhappy—perhaps to be idle and selfish." There is something not quite right in a woman who shuts up her heart from other women.

This may seem to be telling you what you already know, and

bidding you do what you are already doing. Well, then, shall we put the matter another way? Make such friendships as you will look back upon with pleasure in later life, and be loyal and true to your friends, not going from one to another.

> The friends thou hast, and their adoption tried,
> Grapple them to thy soul with hooks of steel;
> But do not dull thy palm with entertainment
> Of each new-hatched, unfledged comrade.

And do not expect more of them than friends can give, or weary them with demands for sympathy; and do not let the womanliness of friendship be impaired by any silliness or sentimentalism; or allow hearty and genial good-will to degenerate into vulgarity and noise.

And as was once truly said, friendship perhaps appears best, as it did in St. Paul, in his manner of rebuking those who had erred, "transferring their faults in a figure to Apollos and to himself." "No one knew how to speak the truth in love like him."

It has been said of Romans xii.: "What rule of manners can be better than this chapter?" "She that giveth, let her do it with simplicity"; that is, let us do our acts of Nursing and kindness as if we did not make much of them, as unto the Lord and not to men. "Like-minded one towards another"; that is, we should have the same thoughts and feelings with others. "Rejoicing with them that rejoice, and weeping with them that weep"; going out of ourselves and entering into the thoughts of others.

And have we St. Paul's extraordinary regard for the feelings of others? He was never too busy to think of these. "If meat make my brother to offend, I will eat no more meat while the world standeth," he says, though he well knew such scruples were really superstitions. If the spirit of these words could find a way to our women's hearts, we might be able to say, "See how these Christians (Nurses) love one another!"

Then the courtesy we owe, one woman to another: "for the

happiness and the good" of our work and our School is not simply "made up of great duties and virtues, nor the evil of the opposite." But both seem to consist also in a number of small particulars, which, small as they are, have a great effect on the tone and character of our School, introducing light or darkness into the "Home," sweetness or bitterness into our intercourse with one another.

And, as to our Wards: Christ, we may be sure, did not lose authority, or dignity and refinement, "even in the company of publicans and harlots," just as we may observe in the Wards, that there are a few of us whose very refinement makes them do the coarsest and roughest things there with simplicity. A Sister of ours once remarked this of one of her Probationers (who was not a lady in the common sense of the word, but she was the truest gentlewoman in Christ's sense), that she was too refined (most people would have said, to do the indelicate work of the Wards, but *she* said) to see indelicacy in doing the nastiest thing; and so did it all well, without thinking of herself, or that men's eyes were upon her. That is real dignity—the dignity which Christ had— on which no man can intrude, yet combined with the greatest gentleness and simplicity of life.

And let me say a word about self-denial: because, as we all know, there can be no real Nursing without self-denial. We know the story of the Roman soldier, above fourteen hundred years ago, who, entering a town in France with his regiment, saw a sick man perishing with cold by the wayside—there were no Hospitals then—and, having nothing else to give, drew his sword, cut his own cloak in half, and wrapped the sick man in half his cloak.

It is said that a dream visited him, in which he found himself admitted into heaven, and Christ saying, "Martin hath clothed me with this garment": the dream, of course, being a remembrance of the verse, "When saw we thee sick or in prison, and came unto thee?" and of the answer, "Inasmuch as ye have done it unto one of the least of these my brethren, ye have done it unto me." But whether the story of the dream be true or not, this Roman soldier, converted to Christianity, became afterwards one of the greatest bishops of the early ages, Martin of Tours.

We are not called upon to feed our patients with our own dinners, or to dress them with our own clothes. We are comfortable, and cannot make ourselves uncomfortable on purpose. But we can learn Sick Cookery for our Patients, we can give up spending our money in foolish dressy ways, and thus squandering what we ought to lay by for ourselves or our families.

On one of the severest winter days in the late war between France and Germany, an immense detachment, many thousands, of wretched French prisoners were passing through the poorest streets of one of the largest and poorest German towns on the way to the prisoners' camp. Every door in this poor "East End" opened; not one remained closed; and out of every door came a poor German woman, carrying in her hand the dinner or supper she was cooking for herself, her husband, or children; often all she had in the house was in her hands. And this she crammed into the hands of the most sickly-looking prisoner as he passed by, often into his mouth, as he sank down exhausted in the muddy street. And the good-natured German escort, whose business it was to bring these poor French to their prison, turned away their heads, and let the women have their way, though it was late, and they were weary too. Before the prisoners had been the first hour in their prison, six had lain down in the straw and died. But how many lives had been saved that night by the timely food of these good women, giving all they had, not of their abundance, but of their poverty, God only knows, not we. This was told by an Englishman who was by and saw it; one of our own "Aid Committee."

And at a large German station, which almost all the prisoners' trains passed through, a lady went every night during all that long, long, dreadful winter, and for the whole night, to feed, and warm, and comfort, and often to receive the last dying words of the miserable French prisoners, as they arrived in open trucks, some frozen to the bottom, some only as the dead, others to die in the station, all half-clad and starving. Some had been nine days and nights in these open trucks; many had been twenty-four hours without food. Night after night as these long, terrible trainsful dragged their slow length into the station, she kneeled on its pavement, supporting the dying heads, receiving their last messages to their mothers; pouring wine or hot milk down the throats of the sick; dressing the frost-bitten limbs; and, thank God, saving many. Many were carried to the prisoners' hospital in the town, of whom about two-thirds recovered. Every bit of linen she had went in this way. She herself contracted incurable ill-health during these fearful nights. But thousands were saved by her means.

She is my friend.[6] She came and saw me here after this; and it is from her lips I heard the story. Smallpox and typhus raged among the prisoners, most of whom were quite boys. Many were wounded; half were frost-bitten. Sometimes they would snatch at all she brought; but sometimes they would turn away their dying heads from the tempting hot wine, and gasp out, "Thank you, madam; give it to *him*, who wants it more than I." Or, "I'm past help; love to mother."

We have not to give of our own to *our* sick. But shall we the less give them our all—that is, all our hearts and minds? and reasonable service?

Suppose we dedicated this "School" to Him, to the Divine Charity and Love which said, "Inasmuch as ye do it unto one of the least of these my brethren" (and He calls all our patients—all of us, His brothers and sisters) "ye do it unto me"—oh, what a "Kingdom of Heaven" this might be! Then, indeed, the dream of Martin of Tours, the soldier and Missionary-Bishop, would have come true!

May I take this opportunity of saying what I think really very much concerns us? First of all, that you have, or might have, directly and indirectly, a great deal to do with maintaining a supply of good candidates to this School. You know whether you have been happy here or not; you know whether you have had opportunities given you here of training and self-improvement. Many, very many of our old Matrons and Nurses have told me that their time as probationers with us was "the happiest time of their lives." It *might* be so with all, though perhaps all do not think so now.

It is in your power to assist the School most materially in obtaining fresh and worthy recruits. There is hardly one of you who has not friends or acquaintances of her own. You *ought* to advertise us. We ought not to have to put one advertisement in the newspapers. If you think this is a worthy life, why do you not bring others to it? I tried to do my part. When Agnes Jones died, though my heart was breaking, I put an article in *Good Words*, such as I knew she would have wished, in all but the mention of herself; and for years her dear memory brought aspirants to the work in our Schools, or others' Schools.

To reform the Nursing of all the Hospitals and Workhouse Infirmaries in the world, and to establish District Nursing among the sick poor at home, too, as at Liverpool—is this not an object most worthy of the co-operation of all civilised people?

In the last ten years, thank God, numerous Training Schools for Nurses have grown up, resolved to unite in putting a stop to such a thing as drunken, immoral, and inefficient Nursing. But all make the same complaint; while the outcry of "employment for women" continues, why does not this most womanly employment for all good women become more sought after? I hope to hear that my old friends in St. Thomas' have each done their part; and I feel quite sure that if it is once placed before them, as a thing they ought to do, they will be found in the front.

You who are assembled in this room, and who are each connected with some circle, directly or indirectly, may do a good work for the civilisation of the Workhouses and Hospitals of the world. If you inform yourselves on the subject, and if you set yourselves to work, to deal with it, as we do with any other great evil that tortures helpless people, you will be able to act directly upon your friends outside, and ultimately get up an amount of public opinion among women capable of becoming Nurses, which will be of the greatest possible aid to our efforts in improving Hospital and Workhouse Nursing. Every one can help—every one—better than if she were a "newspaper," better than if she were a "public meeting." I believe that within a few years you can make it a thing that will be a disgrace to any Hospital or even Workhouse to be suspected of bad Nursing, or to any district (in towns, at any rate) not to have a good District Nurse to nurse the sick poor at home.

Those who have made the right use of all the training that came in their way in this School, if they would write to their own homes for the information of their friends outside, an immense help on its way could be given to the work we have all so much at heart. And I look upon it as a certainty that you will each be able, in one way or another, whether purposely or almost unconsciously, to take a great part in reforming the Hospital and Workhouse Nursing systems of our country, perhaps of our colonies and dependencies, and perhaps of the world.

May I pay ourselves even the least little compliment, as to our being a little less conceited than last year? Were we not as conceited in 1872 as it was possible to be? You shall tell. Are we, in 1873, rather less so? And, without having any one particularly in my head—for what I am going to ask is in fact a truism—is not our conceit always in exact proportion to our ignorance? For those who really know something know how little it is.

Would that this could be a "secret" among us! But, unfortunately, is not our name "up" and "abroad" for conceit? And has it not even been said ("tell it not in Gath"): "And these conceited 'Nightingale' women scarcely know how to read and write?"

Now let no one look to see our blushes. But shall we not get rid of this which makes us ridiculous as fast as we can?

But enough of this joke; let us be serious, remembering that the greatest trust which is committed to any woman of us all is, *herself*; and that she is living in the presence of God as well as of her fellow-women.

To know whether we know our Nursing business or not is a great result of training; and to think that we know it when we do *not* is as great a proof of want of training.

The world, more especially the Hospital world, is in such a hurry, is moving so fast, that it is too easy to slide into bad habits before we are aware. And it is easier still to let our year's training slip away without forming any real plan of training ourselves.

For, after all, all that any training is to do for us is: to teach us how to train ourselves, how to observe for ourselves, how to think out things for ourselves. Don't let us allow the first week, the second week, the third week to pass by—I will not say in idleness, but in bustle. Begin, for instance, at once making notes of your cases. From the first moment you see a case, you can observe it. Nay, it is one of the first things a Nurse is strictly called upon to do: to observe her sick. Mr. Croft has taught you how to take notes; and you have now, every one of you, two leisure times a week to work up your notes.

But give but one-quarter of an hour a *day* to jot down, even in words which no one can understand but yourself, the progress or change of two or three individual cases, not to forget or confuse them. You can then write them out at your two leisure times. To those who have not much education, I am sure that our kind Home Sister, or the Special Probationer in the same Ward, or nearest in any way, will give help. The race is not always to the swift, nor the battle to the strong; and "line upon line"—*one* line every day—in the steady, observing, humble Nurse has often won the race over the smarter "genius" in what constitutes real Nursing. But few of us women seriously think of improving our own mind or character *every day*. And this is fatal to our improving in Nursing. We do not calculate the future by our experience of the past. What right have we to expect that, if we have not improved during the last six months, we shall during the next six? Then, we do not allow for the changes which circumstances make in us—the being put on Staff duty, when we certainly shall not have more time, but less, for improving ourselves, or the growing older or more feeble in health. We believe that we shall always have the same powers or opportunities for learning our business which we now have. Our time of training slips away in this unimproving manner. And when a woman begins to see how many things might have been better in her, she is too old to change, or it is too late, too late. And she confesses to herself, or oftener she does not confess—"How all her life she had been in the wrong."

We are all of us, as we believe, passing into an unknown world, of which this is only a part. We have been here a year, or part of a year. What are we making of our own lives? Are we where we were a year ago? Or are we fitter for that work of after-life which we have undertaken?

Do our faults, and weaknesses, and vanities, tend to diminish? Or are we still listless, inefficient, slow, bustling, conceited, unkind, hard judges of others, instead of helping them where we can? There is no greater softener of hard judgments than is the trying to help the person whom we so judge, as I can tell from my own experience; and in this you will tell me whether we have been deficient to each other. There is a true story told of Captain Marryat when a boy; that he jumped overboard to save an older midshipman who had made the boy's life a misery to him by his filthy cruelties. And the boy Marryat wrote home to his mother "that he loved this midshipman now—and wasn't it lucky that his life was saved—even better than his own darling mother."

Do we keep before our minds constantly the sense of our duty here, of our duty to others—Nurses, Sisters, Matron—as well as to ourselves, our fellow Probationers, and our Home Sister, and to the whole School of which we are members?

If we thought of this more, we might hope to attain that quiet mind and self-control, which is the "liberty" spoken of by St. Paul. We might learn how truly to use and enjoy both our fellow Probationers, and this Home and our School, if we were more anxious about following the example of Christ than about the opinion of our "world." "We are the 'world,' which we often seem to think includes every one but *us*."

But few comparatively have the power of disengaging themselves, even in thought, from those about them. They take the view of their own set. If it is the fashion to conceal, they conceal; if to carry tales, they carry tales. There are a few who never allow themselves to speak against others, and exercise such a kind of authority as to prevent others being spoken against in their hearing. These are the "peacemakers" of whom Christ speaks. These are they who keep a Home or Institution together, and seem more than any others in this our little world to bear the image of Christ until His coming again.

Do we ever do things because they are right, without regard to our own credit? When we ask ourselves only "What is right?" or (which is the same question), "What is the will of God?" then we are truly entering His "kingdom." We are no longer grovelling among the opinions of men and women. We can see God in all things, and all things in God, the Eternal Father shining through the accidents of our lives—which sometimes shake us more, though less conspicuous, than the accidents we see brought into our Surgical Wards—the accidents of the characters of those under whom we are placed, and of our own inner life.

One of the greatest missionaries that ever was, wrote more than 300 years ago to his pupils and fellow-missionaries:

"Self-knowledge"—(the knowledge by which we see ourselves in God)—"self-knowledge is the nurse of confidence in God. It is from distrust of ourselves that confidence in God is born. This will be the way for us to gain that true interior lowliness of mind which, in all places, and especially here, is far more necessary than you think. I warn you also not to let the good opinion which men have of you be too much of a pleasure to you, unless perhaps in order that you may be the more ashamed of yourselves on that account. It is that which leads people to neglect themselves, and this negligence, in many cases, upsets, *as by a kind of trick*, all that lowliness of which I speak, and puts conceit and arrogance in its place. And thus so many do not see for a long time how much they have lost, and gradually lose all care for piety, and all tranquillity of mind, and thus are always troubled and anxious, finding no comfort either from without or within themselves."

"Come unto me, all ye that labour and are heavy laden," says our Lord, "and I will give you rest." But He adds immediately who those are to whom He will give this "rest" or quietness of mind—namely those, who, like Himself, are "meek and lowly of heart."

These words may seem in a Hospital life "like dreams." But they are not dreams if we take them for the spirit of our School and the rule of our Nursing. "To practise them, to feel them, to make them our own," this is not far from the "kingdom of Heaven" in a Hospital.

Pray for me, as I do for you, that "piety" and a "quiet mind"—but these always and only in the strenuous effort to *press forwards*—may be ours.

FLORENCE NIGHTINGALE.

III

July 23rd, 1874.

Another year has passed over us, my dear friends. There have been many changes among us. We have each of us tasted somewhat more of the discipline of life. To some of us it may have been very bitter; to others, let us hope, not so. By all, let us trust, it has been put to heroic uses.

"Heroic?" I think I hear you say; "can there be much of 'heroic' in washing porringers and making beds?"

I once heard a man (he is dead now) giving a lesson to some poor orphan girls in an Orphan Asylum. Few things, I think, ever struck me so much, or them. It was on the "heroic virtues." It went into the smallest particulars of thrift, of duty, of love and kindness; and he ended by asking them how they thought such small people as themselves could manage to practise those great virtues. A child of seven put up its little nib and chirped out: "Please, my lord, we might pick up pins when we don't like to." That showed she understood his lesson.

His lesson was not exactly fitted to us, but we may all fit it to ourselves.

This night, if we are inclined to make a noise on the stairs, or to linger in each other's rooms, shall we go quietly to bed, alone with God? Some of you yourselves have told me that you could get better day sleep in the Night Nurses' Dormitory than in your own "Home." Is there such loud laughing and boisterous talking in the daytime, going upstairs to your rooms, that it disturbs any one who is ill, or prevents those who have been on night duty from getting any sleep?

Is that doing what you would be done by—loving your neighbour as yourselves, as our Master told us?

Do you think it is we who invent the duty "Quiet and orderly," or is it He?

If our uniform dress is not what we like, shall we think of our Lord, whose very garments were divided by the soldiers? (But I always think how much more becoming is our uniform than any other dress I see.)

If there is anything at table that we don't like, shall we take it thankfully, remembering Who had to ask a poor woman for a drink of water?

Shall we take the utmost pains to be perfectly regular and punctual to all our hours—going into the wards, coming out of the wards, at meals, etc.?

And if we are unavoidably prevented, making an apology to the Home Sister, remembering what has been written about those who are in authority over us? Or do we think a few minutes of no consequence in coming from or going to the wards?

Do we carefully observe our Rules?

If we *are* what is printed at the top of our Duties, viz.:

Trustworthy,
Punctual,
Quiet and orderly,
Cleanly and neat,
Patient, cheerful, and kindly,

we scarcely need any other lesson but what explains these to us.

Trustworthy: that is, faithful.

Trustworthy when we have no one by to urge or to order us. "Her lips were never opened but to speak the truth." Can that be said of us?

Trustworthy, in keeping our soul in our hands, never excited, but always ready to lift it up to God; unstained by the smallest flirtation, innocent of the smallest offence, even in thought.

Trustworthy, in doing our work as faithfully as if our superiors were always near us.

Trustworthy, in never prying into one another's concerns, but ever acting behind another's back as one would to her face.

Trustworthy, in avoiding every word that could injure, in the smallest degree, our patients, or our companions, who are our neighbours, remembering how St. Peter says that God made us *all* "stewards of grace one to another."

How can we be "stewards of grace" to one another? By giving the "grace" of our good example to all around us. And how can we become "untrustworthy stewards" to one another? By showing ourselves lax in our habits, irregular in our ways, not doing as we should do if our superiors were by. "Cripple leads the way." Shall the better follow the worse?

It has happened to me to hear some of you say—perhaps it has happened to us all—"Indeed, I only did what I saw done."

How glorious it would be if "only doing what we saw done"

always led us right!

A master of a great public school once said that he could trust his whole school, because he could trust every single boy in it. Oh, could God but say that He can trust this Home and Hospital because He can trust every woman in it! Let us try this—every woman to work as though success depended on herself. Do you know that, in this great Indian Famine, every Englishman has worked as if success depended on himself? And in saving a population as large as that of England from death by starvation, do you not think that we have achieved the greatest victory we ever won in India? Suppose we work thus for this Home and Hospital.

Oh, my dear friends, how terrible it will be to any one of us, some day, to hear another say, that she only did what she saw us do, if that was on the "road that leadeth to destruction"!

Or taking it another way, how delightful—how delightful to have set another on her journey to heaven by our good example; how terrible to have delayed another on her journey to heaven by our bad example!

There is an old story—nearly six hundred years old—when a ploughboy said to a truly great man, whose name is known in history, that he "advised" him "always to live in such a way that those who had a good opinion of him might never be disappointed."

The great man thanked him for his advice, and—kept it.

If our School has a good name, do we live so that people "may never be disappointed" in its Nurses?

Obedient: not wilful: not having such a sturdy will of our own. Common sense tells us that no training can do us any good, if we are always seeking our own way. I know that some have really sought in dedication to God to give up their own wills to His. For if you enter this Training School, is that not in effect a promise to Him to give up your own way for that way which you are taught?

Let us not question so much. You *must* know that things have been thought over and arranged for your benefit. You are not bound to think us always right: perhaps you can't. But are *you* more likely to be right? And, at all events, you know you *are* right, if you choose to enter our ways, to submit yours to them.

In a foreign Training School, I once heard a most excellent pastor, who was visiting there, say to a nurse: "Are you *dis*couraged?—say rather, you are *dis*obedient: they always mean the same thing." And I thought how right he was. And, what is more, the Nurse thought so too; and she was not "discouraged" ever after, because she gave up being "disobedient."

"Every one for herself" ought to have no footing here: and these strong wills of ours God will teach. If we do not let Him teach us here, He will teach us by some sterner discipline hereafter—teach our wills to bend first to the will of God, and then to the reasonable and lawful wills of those among whom our lot is cast.

I often say for myself, and I have no doubt you do, that line of the hymn:

Tell me, Thou yet wilt chide, Thou canst not spare, O Lord, Thy chastening rod.

Let Him reduce us to His discipline before it is too late. If we "kick against the pricks," we can only pray that He will give us more "pricks," till we cease to "kick." And it is a proof of His fatherly love, and that He has not given us up, if He does.

For myself, I can say that I have never known what it was, since I can remember anything, not to have "prickly" discipline, more than any one knew of; and I hope I have not "kicked."

To return to *Trustworthiness.*

Most of you, on leaving the Home, go first on night duty. Now there is nothing like night duty for trying our trustworthiness. A year hence you will tell me whether you have felt any temptation not to be quite honest in reporting cases the next morning to your Sister or Nurse: that is, to say you have observed when you have not observed; to slur over things in your report, which, for aught you know, may be of consequence to the patient: to slur over things in your work because there is no one watching you: no one but God.

It has indeed been known that the Night Nurse had stayed in the kitchen to talk; but we may trust such things will not happen again.

And, for all, let us *all* say this word for ourselves: everything gets toppled over if we don't make it a matter of conscience, a matter of reckoning between ourselves and our God. That is the only safeguard of real *trustworthiness*. If we treat it as a mere matter of business, of success in our career in life, never shall we give anything but eye-service, never shall we be really trustworthy.

Orderly: Let us never waste anything, even pins or paper, as some do, by beginning letters or resolutions, or "cases," which they never take the trouble to finish.

Cheerful and Patient: Let us never wish for more than is necessary, and be cheerful when what we should like is sometimes denied us, as it may be some day; or when people are unkind, or we are disregarded by those we love: remembering Him whose attendants at His death were mocking soldiers.

I assure you, my friends, that if we can practise those "duties" faithfully, we are practising the "heroic virtues."

Patient, cheerful, and kindly: Now, is it being patient, cheerful, and kindly to be so only with those who are so to us? For, as St. Peter tells us, even ungodly people do that. But if we can do good to some one who has done us ill, oh, what a privilege that is! And even God will thank us for it, the Apostle says. Let us be kindest to the impatient and unkindly.

Now let me tell you of two Nurses whom we knew.

One was a lady, with just enough to live upon, who took an old widow to nurse into her house: recommended to her by her minister. One day she met him and reproached him. Why? Because the old widow was "too good"; "*any*body could nurse *her.*" Presently a grumbling old woman, never contented with anything anybody did, who thought she was never treated well enough, and that she never had "her due," was found. And this old woman the lady took into her house and nursed till she died;

because, she said, nobody else liked to do anything for her, and *she* did. That was something like kindness, for there is no great kindness in doing good to any one who is grateful and thanks us for it.

But my other story is something much better still.

A poor Nurse, who had been left a widow, with nothing to live upon but her own earnings, inquired for some *tedious children* to take care of. As you may suppose, there was no difficulty in finding this article. And from that day, for twenty years, she never had less than two, three, or four orphans with her, and sometimes five, whom she brought up as her own, training them for service. She taught them domestic work, for she herself went out to service at nine years old. She never had any difficulty in finding places for them, and for twenty years she had thus a succession of children. But she taught them something better.

She taught them that they had "nothing but their character to depend upon." "I tell them," she said, "it was all I had myself; God helps girls that watch over themselves. If a girl isn't made to feel this early, it's hard afterwards to make her feel it."

These girls, so brought up, turned out much better than those brought up in most large Union schools, for asylums are not like homes. Of the children whom Nurse took in, one was a girl of such bad habits and such a mischief-maker that no one else could manage her. But Nurse did. She soon found she could not refuse boys. One was a boy of fourteen, just out of prison for bad ways, whom she took and reclaimed, and who became as good a boy as can be. These are only two specimens.

They called her "Mother." And God, she used to say, gave them to her as her own. You will ask how she supported them. The larger number of them she supported by taking in washing, by charing one day a week, and bye and bye, by taking in journeymen as lodgers. Now and then a lady would pay for an orphan. Once she took in a sailor's five motherless children for 5s. a week from the father: but she has taken in apprentices as lodgers, whose own fathers could not afford to keep them for their wages.

All this time she washed for a poor sick Irishwoman, who never gave her any thanks but that "the clothes were not well washed, nor was anything done as it ought to be done." Yet she took in this woman's child of two years old as her own, till the father came back, when he gave up drink and claimed it.

Every Friday she gave her earnings to some poor women, who bought goods with the money, which they sold again in the market on Saturday, and returned her money to her on Saturday night. She said she never lost a penny by this: and it kept several old women going.

She must have been a capital manager, you will say. Well, till she took in lodgers, she lived in a cellar which she painted with her own hands, and kept as clean as a new pin. Afterwards she let her cellar for 2s. a week, though she might have got 2s. 6d. or 3s. a week for it, because, she said, "the poor should not be hard on one another." Milk she never tasted; meat seldom, and then she always stewed, never roasted it. She lived on potatoes, and potato pie was the luxury of herself and children.

On Sundays she filled her pot of four gallons and made broth: sometimes for six or eight poor old women besides her own family, as she called her orphans. *These* must be satisfied with what she provided, little or much. She never let them touch what was sent her for her patients. Sometimes good things were sent her, which she always gave to sick neighbours; yet she has been accused of keeping for herself nice things sent to her care for others. She never owed a penny, for all her charity.

If this Nurse has not practised the "heroic virtues," who has?

I mentioned this Nurse merely as an instance of one who literally fulfilled the precept to "do good" to them that "despitefully use you": to be "patient, cheerful, and kindly." There is no time to tell you how she was left a widow with two infants and a blind and insane mother, whom she kept till doctors compelled her to put her mother into a lunatic asylum: how one of her sons was a sickly cripple, whom she nursed till he died, working by day and sitting up with him at night for years: how the other boy was insane, and ran away: how, to ease her broken mother's heart, she returned to sick-nursing, chiefly among the poor, nursed through two choleras, till her health broke down, and, by way of taking care of herself, then took up the "tedious" orphan system, which she never ceased. She felt, she said, as if she were doing something then for her "own dear boy." As soon as she lived in a poor house of four rooms and an attic, she has had as many as ten carpenters' men of a night, who had nowhere but the public-house to go to. She gave them a good fire, borrowed a newspaper for them, and made one read aloud. They brought her sixpence a week, and she laid it all out in supper for them, and cooked it. She gave the only good pair of shoes she had to one of these, because "he must go to work decent!"

She was a famous sick cook, often carrying home fish-bones to stew them for the sick, who seldom thanked her; and the remains of damsons and currants, to boil over again as a drink for fever patients: who sometimes accused her of keeping back things sent for them.

"How much more the Lord has borne from me," she used to say.

And of children she used to say: "We never can train up a child in the way it should go till we take it in our arms, as Jesus did, and feel: 'Of such is the kingdom of heaven'; and that there is a 'heavenly principle' (a 'little angel,' I think she said) in each child to be trained up in it."

She said she had learnt this from the master in a factory where she had once nursed.

(How little he knew that he had been one means of forming this heroic Nurse.)

And now I have a word for the Ladies, and a word for the Nurse-Probationers. Which shall come first?

Do the ladies follow up their intellectual privileges? Or, are they lazy in their hours of study? Do they cultivate their powers of expression in answering Mr. Croft's examinations?

Ought they not to look upon themselves as future leaders—as those who will have to train others? And to bear this in mind during the whole of their year's training, so as to qualify themselves for being so? It is not just getting through the year anyhow, without being blamed. For the year leaves a stamp on everybody—this for the Nurses as well as the Ladies—and once gone can never be regained.

To the Special Probationers may I say one more word?

Do we look enough into the importance of giving ourselves thoroughly to study in the hours of study, of keeping careful *Notes of Lectures*, of keeping notes of all type cases, and of cases interesting from not being type cases, so as to improve our powers of observation—all essential *if we are in future to have charge*? Do we keep in view the importance of helping ourselves to understand these cases by reading at the time books where we can find them described, and by listening to the remarks made by Physicians and Surgeons in going round with their Students? (Take a sly note afterwards, when nobody sees, in order to have a correct remembrance.)

So shall we do everything in our power to become proficient, not only in knowing the symptoms and what is to be done, but in knowing the "Reason Why" of such symptoms, and *why* such and such a thing is done; and so on, till we can some day TRAIN OTHERS *to know the "reason why."*

Many say: "We have no time; the Ward work gives us no time."

But it is so easy to degenerate into a mere drudgery about the Wards, when we have goodwill to do it, and are fonder of practical work than of giving ourselves the trouble of learning the "reason why." Take care, or the Nurses, some of them, will catch you up.

Take ten minutes a day in the Ward to jot down things, and write them out afterwards: come punctually *from* your Ward to have time for doing so. *It is far better to take these ten minutes to write your cases or to jot down your recollections in the Ward than to give the same ten minutes to bustling about.* I am sure the

Sisters would help you to get this time if you asked them: and also to *leave* the Ward punctually.

And do you not think this a religious duty?

Such observations are a religious meditation: for is it not the best part of religion to imitate the benevolence of God to man? And how can you do this—in this your calling especially—if you do not thoroughly understand your calling? And is not every study to do this a religious contemplation?

Without it, *May you not potter and cobble about the patients without ever once learning the reason of what you do, so as to be able to train others?*

(I do not say anything about the "cards," for I take it for granted that you can read them easily.)

Our dear Matron, who is always thinking of arranging for us, is going to have a case-paper with printed headings given to you, and to keep this correctly ought to be a mere every-day necessity, and a very easy one, for you.

2. And for the Nurses:

They are placed, perhaps here only, on a footing of equality with educated gentlewomen. Do they show their appreciation of this by thinking, "We are as good as they"? Or, by obedience and respect, and trying to profit by the superior education of the gentlewomen?

Both we have known; we have known Nurse-Probationers who took the Ladies "under their protection" in saving them the harder work, and the Ladies have given them the full return back in helping them in their education.

And we have known—very much the reverse.

Also, do the Nurse-Probationers take advantage of their opportunities, in the excellent classes given them by the Home Sister, in keeping diaries and some cases?

Very few of the Nurse-Probationers have taken notes of Mr. Croft's Lectures at all; it is not fair to Mr. Croft to give him people who do not benefit by his instruction.

3. And I have another word to say:

Are there parties in our Home?

Could we but be *not* so tenacious of our own interests, but look at the thing in a larger way!

Is there a great deal of canvassing and misinterpreting Sisters and Matron and other authorities? every little saying and doing of theirs? talking among one another about the superiors (and then finding we were all wrong when we came to know them better)?

We must all of us know, without being told, that we cannot be trained at all, if in training this will of our own is not kept under.

Do not question so much. Does not a spirit of criticism go with ignorance? Are some of you in all the "opposition of irresponsibility"? Some day, when you are yourselves responsible, you will know what I mean.

Now could not the Ladies help the Nurse-Probationers in this: (1) in never themselves criticising; and (2) in saying a kindly word to check it when it is done?

Let me tell you a true story about this.

In a large college, questions—about things which the students could but imperfectly understand in the conduct of the college—had become too warm. The superintendent went into the hall one morning, and after complimenting the young men on their studies, he said: "This morning I heard two of the porters, while at their work, take up a Greek book lying on my table; one tried to read it, and the other declared it ought to be held upside down to be read. Neither could agree which *was* upside down, but both thought themselves quite capable of arguing about Greek, though neither could read it. They were just coming to fisticuffs, when I sent the two on different errands."

Not a word was added: the students laughed and retired, but they understood the moral well enough, and from that day there were few questions or disputes about the plans and superiors of the college, or about their own obedience to rules and discipline.

Do let us think of the two porters squabbling whether the Greek book was to be read upside down, when we feel inclined to

175

be questioning about "things too high for us."

We are constantly making mistakes in our judgment of our little world. We fancy that we have been harshly treated or misunderstood. Or we cannot bear our fellow-Probationers to laugh at us.

Believe me, there will come a time when all such troubles will simply seem ridiculous to us, and we shall be unable to imagine how we could ever have been the victims of them. (One of your number told me this herself. She has left St. Thomas' for another post.) Let us not brood or sentimentalise over them. They should be met in a common-sense way. How much of our time has been spent in grieving over these trifles, how little in the real sorrow for sin, the real struggle for improvement.

4. As for obedience to rules and our superiors: "True obedience," said one of the most efficient people who ever lived, "obeys not only the command, but also the intention" of those who have a right to command us. Of course, this is a truism: the thing is, *how to do it.* As it is a struggle, it requires a brave and intrepid spirit, which helps us to rise above trifles and look to God, and His leadings for us. Oh, when death comes, how sorry we shall be to have watched others so much and ourselves so little; to have dug so much in the field of others' consciences and left our own fallow! What should we say of a "Leopold" Nurse who should try to nurse in "Edward" Ward, and neglect her own "Leopold"? Well, that is what we do. Or who should wash her patients' hands and not her own?

It is of ourselves and not of others that we must give an account. Let us look to our own consciences as we do to our own hands, to see if they are dirty.

We take care of our dress, but do we take care of our words?

It is a very good rule to say and do nothing but what we can offer to God. Now we cannot offer Him backbiting, petty scandal, misrepresentation, flirtation, injustice, bad temper, bad thoughts, jealousy, murmuring, complaining. Do we ever think that we bear the responsibility of all the harm we do in this way?

Look at that busybody who fidgets, gossips, makes a bustle, always wanting to domineer, always thinking of herself, as if she wanted to tell the sun to get out of her way and let her light the world in its place, as the proverb says.

And when we might do all our actions and say all our words as unto God!

So many imperfections; so many thoughts of self-love; so many selfish satisfactions that we mix with our best actions! And when we might offer them all to God. What a pity!

5. One word more for the Ladies, or those who will have to train and look after others.

What must she be who is to be a Ward or "Home" Sister?

We see her in her nobleness and simplicity: being, not seeming: without name or reward in this world: "clothed" in her "righteousness" merely, as the Psalms would say, *not* in her dignity: often having no gifts of money, speech, or strength: but never preferring seeming to being.

And if she rises still higher, she will find herself, in some measure, like the Great Example in Isaiah liii., bearing the sins and sorrows of others as if they were her own: her counsels often "despised and rejected," yet "opening not her mouth" to be angry: "led as a lamb to the slaughter."

She who rules best is she who loves best: and shows her love not by foolish indulgence to those of whom she is in charge, but by taking a real interest in them for their own sakes, and in their highest interests.

Her firmness must never degenerate into nervous irritability. And for this end let me advise you when you become Sisters, always to take your exercise time out of doors, your monthly day out, and your annual holiday.

Be a judge of the work of others of whom you are in charge, not a detective: your mere detective "is wonderful at suspicion and discovery," but is often at fault, foolishly imagining that every one is bad.

The Head-Nurse must have been tested in the refiner's fire, as the prophets would say: have been tried by many tests: and have come out of them stainless, in full command of herself and her principles: never losing her temper.

She never nurses well till she ceases to command for the sake of commanding, or for her own sake at all: till she nurses only for the sakes of those who are nursed. This is the highest exercise of self-denial; but without it the ruin of the nursing, of the charge, is sure to come.

Have we ever known such a Nurse?

She must be just, not unjust.

Now justice is the perfect order by which every woman does her own business, and injustice is where every woman is doing another's business. This is the most obvious of all things: and for that very reason has never been found out. Injustice is the habit of being a busybody and doing another woman's business, which tries to rule and ought to serve: this is the unjust Nurse.

Prudence is doing your nursing most perfectly: aiming at the perfect in everything: this is the "seeking God and His righteousness" of the Scriptures.

And must not each of us be a Saviour, rather than a ruler: each in our poor measure? Did the Son of God try to rule? Oh, my friends, do not scold at women: they will be of another mind if they are "gently entreated" and learn to know you. Who can hate a woman who loves them? Or be jealous of one who has no jealousy? Who can squabble with one who never squabbles? It is example which converts your patients, your ward-maids, your fellow-Nurses or charges: it is example which converts the world.

And is not the Head-Nurse or Sister there, not that she may do as she likes, but that she should serve all for the common good of all? The one worst maxim of all for a future Matron, Sister, or Nurse is "to do as I like": that *is* disorder, not rule. It is giving power to evil.

Those who rule must not be those who are desirous to rule.

She who is best fitted is often the least inclined to rule: but if the necessity is laid upon her, she takes it up as a message from

God. And she must no longer live in her own thoughts, making a heaven or hell of her own. For if she does not make a heaven for others, her charge will soon become something else.

She must never become excited: and therefore I do impress upon you regularity and punctuality, and never to get hurried. Those often get most excited who are least in earnest. She who is fierce with her Nurses, her patients, or her ward-maid, is not truly above them: she is below them: and, although a harsh ward-mistress to her patients or Nurses, has no real superiority over them.

There is no impudence like that of ignorance. Each night let us come to a knowledge of ourselves before going to rest: as the Psalm says: "Commune with your own heart upon your bed, *and be still.*" Is it possible that we who live among the sick and dying can be satisfied not to make *friends* with *God* each night?

The future Sister should be neither mistress nor servant, but the *friend* of every woman under her. If she is mistress of others when she is not mistress of herself, her jealous, faithless temper grows worse with command (oh, let not this be the case with any of us!)—wanting everything of everybody, yet not knowing how to get it of anybody. Always in fear, confusion, suspicion, and distraction, she becomes more and more faithless, envious, unrighteous, the cause of wretchedness to herself and others. She who has no control over herself, who cannot master her own temper, how can she be placed over others, to control them through the better principle? But she who is the most royal mistress of herself is the only woman fit to be in charge.

For this is the whole intention of training, education, supervision, superintendence: to give self-control, to train or nurse up in us a higher principle; and when this is attained, you may go your ways safely into the world.

But she who nurses, and does not nurse up in herself the "infant Christ," who should be born again in us every day, is like an empty syringe—it pumps in only wind.

The future Sister must be not of the governessing but of the

Saviour turn of mind.

Let her reason with the unjust woman who is not intentionally in error. She must know how to give good counsel, which will advise what is best under the circumstances; not making a lament, but finding a cure; regarding *that* only as "bettering" their situation which *makes them better*. She must know and teach "how to refuse the evil and choose the good," as Isaiah says.

She must have an iron sense of truth and right for herself and others, and a golden sense of love and charity for them.

When a future Sister unites the power of command with the power of thought and love, when she can raise herself and others above the commonplaces of a common self without disregarding any of our common feelings, when she can plan and effect any reforms wanted step by step, without trying to precipitate them into a single year or month, neither hasting nor delaying: that is indeed a "Sister."

The future Sister or Head must not see only a little corner of things, her own petty likes and dislikes; she must "lift up her eyes to the hills," as David says. She must know that there is a greater and more real world than her own littlenesses and meannesses. And she must be not only the friend of her Nurses, but also, in her measure, the angel whose mission is to reconcile her Nurses to themselves, to each other, and to God.

Now let us not each of us think how this fits on to her neighbour, but how it fits on to oneself.

Shall I tell you what one of you said to me after I last addressed you?—"Do you think we are missionaries?"

I answer, that you cannot help being missionaries, if you would. There are missionaries for evil as well as for good. Can you help choosing? Must you not decide whether you will be missionaries for good, or whether for evil, among your patients and among yourselves?

And, first, among your patients:

Hospital Nurses have charge of their patients in a way that no other woman has charge; in the first place, no other woman is in charge really of grown-up men. Oh, how careful she ought to be, especially the Night Nurse, to show them what a true woman can be! The acts of a nurse are keenly scrutinised by both old and young patients. If she is not perfectly pure and upright, depend upon it, they know.

Also, a Hospital Nurse is in charge of people in their sick and feeble, anxious and dying hours, when they are singularly alive to impressions. She leaves her stamp upon them, whether she will or no. And this applies almost more to the Night Nurse than to the Day Nurse.

Lastly, if she have children-patients, she is absolutely in charge of these, who come, perhaps for the first and the last time of their lives, under influence.

So many pass by a child without notice. A whole life of happiness or wretchedness may turn upon an act of kindness to it—a good example set it. A poor woman once said of a child of hers under just these circumstances: "The Sister set its face heavenwards: and it never looked back." Do we ever set their faces the other way? The child she spoke of when it was dying actually gave its halfpence, which it had saved for something for itself, for another dying child "who had nobody." I call *that* practising the "heroic virtues," if ever there were such. And that was done under just such an influence as we have been speaking of.

On the other hand, do you know anything in its way more heinous than a Nurse, who to the sick and tiresome child might be like an angel "to set its face heavenward" by her sympathy with it, and who, by her own bad habits or bad temper, by her unfairness, by her unkindness or injustice, by her coarseness or want of uprightness, sets it the other way?

A very good man once said that in each little Hospital patient, he saw not only a soul to be saved, but many other souls that might possibly be committed to this one: for the poor can do so much among one another: do what no others going among them can do. Every child is of the stuff out of which Home Missionaries may be made, such as God chooses from the ranks that have furnished his best recruits.

The Apostles were fishermen and workmen.

David Livingstone was a cotton-mill piecer. In each little pauper waif he saw one destined to carry a godly example (or the reverse) where none but they could carry it—into godless and immoral homes.

We will not repeat here, because we are so fully persuaded of it, that a woman, especially a Nurse, must be a missionary, *not* as a minister or chaplain is, but by the influence of her own character, silent but not unfelt.

It was this, far more than any words, that gave his matchless influence to David Livingstone, whose body, brought upwards of 1500 miles through pathless deserts by his own negro servants— such a heroic feat as Christians never knew before—was buried this spring in Westminster Abbey. Some of us knew him: one of our Probationers was with him and his wife, who died in 1862, and Bishop Mackenzie, at their Mission Station in Africa. He was such a traveller and missionary as we shall never see again perhaps. But what he was in influence each of us may be, if we please, in our little sphere.

A Nurse *is* like a traveller, from the quantity of people who pass before her in the ever-changing wards. And she is like a traveller also in this, that, as Livingstone used to say, either the vices or the virtues of civilisation follow the footsteps of the traveller, and he cannot help it. So they do those of the Nurse. And missioning will be, whether she will or no, the background of her nursing, as it is the background of travelling. The traveller may call himself a missionary or not, as he likes. He *is* one, for good or for evil. So is the Nurse.

Livingstone used to say that we fancy a missionary a man with a Bible in his hand and another in his pack. He then went on to say what a real missionary must be in himself to have influence. And he added: "If I had once been suspected of a single act of want of purity or uprightness the negroes would never have trusted me again. No, not even the least pure or the least upright of the negroes. And any influence of mine would have been gone for ever." What his influence was, even after his death, you know.

Then you must be missionaries, whether you will or no, among one another.

We need only think of the friendships that are made here. Will you be a missionary of good or of evil to your friend? Will you be a missionary of indifference, selfishness, lightness of conduct, self-indulgence? Or a missionary—to her and to your patients—of religious and noble devotion to duty, carried out to the smallest thing?

Will you be a "hero" in your daily work, like the dying child giving its hard-saved halfpence to the yet poorer child?

Livingstone always remembered that a poor old Scotchman on his death-bed had said to him: "Now, lad, make religion the *every-day* business of your life, not a thing of fits and starts; for if you do not, temptation and other things will get the better of you."

Such a Nurse—one who makes religion the "every-day business of her life," *is* a "Missionary," even if she never speak a word. One who does not is a missionary for *evil* and not for good, though she may say many words, have many good texts at the end of her tongue, or, as Livingstone would say, a Bible in her hand and a Bible at her back.

Believe me, who have seen a good deal of the world, we may give you an institution to learn in, but it is You must furnish the "heroic" feeling of doing your duty, doing your best, without which no institution is safe, without which Training Schools are meat without salt. *You* must be our salt, without which civilisation is but corruption, and all churches only dead establishments.

Shall I tell you what one of the most famous clergymen that ever lived said? That, in order to manage people, and especially children, well, it was necessary to speak more of them to God than of God to them. If a famous preacher said that, how much more must a woman?

Another learned clergyman, who was also the best translator of the Bible (in a foreign language), said: "Prayer, rather than speech must be relied upon for the reform of any little irregularities: for only through prayer could the proper moment for speech become known." If a great leader of mankind said that, how much more should a Nurse?

I must end: and what I say now I had better have said: and nothing else.

What are we without God? Nothing.

"Father, glorify Thy name!" How is His name glorified? *We* are His glory, when we follow His ways. Then we are something.

What is the Christian religion? To be like Christ.

And what is it to be like Christ? To be High Church, Low Church, Dissenter, or orthodox? Oh, no. It is: to live for God and have God for our object.

IV

London, *May 26, 1875.*

My dear Friends,—This year my letter to you must needs be short, for I am not able to write much. But good words are always short. The best words that ever were spoken—Christ's words— were the shortest. Would that ours were always the echo of His!

First, then:

What is our one thing needful? To have high principles at the bottom of all. Without this, without having laid our foundation, there is small use in building up our details. That is as if you were to try to nurse without eyes or hands. We know who said, If your foundation is laid in shifting sand, you may build your house, but it will tumble down. But if you build it on solid ground, this is what is called being *rooted and grounded in Christ.*

In the great persecutions in France two hundred years ago (not only of the Protestants, who came over here and settled in Spitalfields, but of all who held the higher and more spiritual religion) a noble woman, who has left her impress on the Christian Church, and who herself endured two hard imprisonments for conscience' sake, would receive no Probationer into her Institution, which was, like ours, for works of Nursing and for the poor, till the Probationer had well considered whether she were really rooted and grounded in God himself, and not in the mere habit of obeying rule and doing her work; whether she could do without the supports of the example and fellowship of a large and friendly community, the sympathy and praise of fellow-workers—all good things in themselves, but which will not carry us through a life like Christ's. And I doubt whether any woman whom God is forming for Himself is not at some time or other of her life tried and tested in this lonely path.

A French Princess, who did well consider, and who was received into the said Institution on these conditions, has left us in writing her experience. And well she showed *where* she was "rooted and grounded" through ten after-years of prison and persecution.

We have not to endure these things. Our lot is cast in gentler times.

But I will tell you an old woman's experience—that I can never remember a time, and that I do not know a work, which so requires to be rooted and grounded in God as ours.

You remember the question in the hymn, "Am I His, or am I not?" If I *am*, this is what is called our "hidden life with Christ in God." We all have a "hidden life" in ourselves, besides our outward working life. If our hidden life is filled with chatter and fancies, our outward working life will be the fruits of it.

"By their *fruits* ye shall know them," Christ says. Christ knows the good Nurse. It is not the good talker whom Christ knows as the good Nurse. If our hidden life *is* "with Christ in God," by its fruits, too, it will be known.

185

What is it to live "with Christ in God"? It is to live in Christ's spirit: forgiving any injuries, real or fancied, from our fellow-workers, from those above us as well as from those below (alas! how small our injuries are that we should talk of forgiving!) thirsting after righteousness, righteousness, *i.e.* doing completely one's duty towards all with whom we have to do, towards God above as well as towards our fellow-nurses, our patients, our matron, home sister, and instructors; fain to be holy as God is holy, perfect as our Father in Heaven is perfect in our hospital and training school; caring for nothing more than for God's will in this His training; careful for our sick and fellow-Nurses more than for ourselves; active, like Christ, in our work; like Christ, meek and lowly in heart in our Wards and "Home"; peacemakers among our companions, which includes the never repeating anything which may do mischief; placing our spirits in the Father's charge. ("I am the Almighty's charge," says the hymn.) *This* is to live a life with Christ in God.

You may have heard of Mr. Wilberforce. He it was who, after a long life of unremitting activity, varied only with disappointment, carried the Abolition of the Slave Trade, one of England's greatest titles to the gratitude of nations. Slavery, as Livingstone said, is the open sore of the world. (Mr. Clarkson and my grandfather were two of his fellow-workers.) Some one asked how Mr. Wilberforce did this, and a man I knew answered, "Because his life was hid with Christ in God."

Never was there a truer word spoken. And if we, when the time comes for us to be in charge of Wards, are enabled to "abolish" anything wrong in them, it can only be in the same way, by our life being hid with Christ in God. And no man or woman will do great things for God, or even small, whose "hidden life" is employed in self-complacency, or in thinking over petty slights, or of what other people are thinking of her.

We have three judges—our God, our neighbour, and ourselves. Our own judgment of ourselves is, perhaps, generally too favourable: our neighbour's judgment of us too unfavourable, except in the case of close friends, who may sometimes spoil each other. Shall we always remember to seek *God's* judgment of us, knowing this, that it will some day find us, whether we seek it or not? *He* knows who is *His* nurse, and who is not.

This is laying the "foundation"; *this* is the "hidden life with Christ in God" for us Nurses. "Keeping up to the mark," as St. Paul says; and nothing else *will* keep us up to the mark in Nursing.

"Neglect nothing; the most trivial action may be performed to ourselves, or performed to God." What a pity that so many actions should be wasted by us Nurses in our Wards and in our "Home," when we might always be doing common things uncommonly well!

Small things *are* of consequence—small things are of *no* consequence; we say this often to ourselves and to each other.

And both these sayings are true.

Every brick is of consequence, every dab of mortar, that it may be as good as possible in building up your house. A chain is no stronger than its weakest link: therefore every link is of consequence. And there can be no "small" thing in Nursing. How often we have seen a Nurse's life wrecked, in its usefulness, by some apparently small fault! Perhaps this is to say that there can be no small things in the nursing service of God.

But in the service of ourselves, oh! how small the things are! Of no consequence indeed. How small they will appear to us all some day!

For what does it profit a Nurse if she gain the whole world to praise her, and lose her own soul in conceit? What does it profit if the judgment of the whole world is for us Nurses, and God's is against us?

It is a real danger, in works like these, when all men praise us. We must then see if we are "rooted and grounded in Christ Himself," to nurse as *He* would have us nurse, as *He* was in God, to do *His* Saviour-work. Am I His, or am I not?

It is a real danger, too, if in works like these we do not uphold

187

the credit of our School. That is *not* bearing fruit. Can we hope, may we hope that, at least, some day, Christ may say even to our Training School, as He did once to His first followers, "Ye are the salt of the earth"? But oh! if we may hope this, let us never forget for one moment the terrible conclusion of that verse.

If we can, in the faintest sense, be called "the salt "of God's nursing world, let us watch, watch, watch, that we may never lose our "savour." One woman, as we well know, may be honoured by God to be "the salt" to purify a whole Ward. One woman may have lost her "savour," and a Ward be left without its "salt," and untold harm done.

We ought to be very much obliged to our kind Medical Instructor for the pains he has taken with us, and to show this by our careful attention. Without this there can be no improvement.

There is a time for all things—a time to be trained, and a time to use our training. And if we have thrown away the year we have here, we can hardly recover it. Besides, what a shame it is to come here, as Probationers, at considerable cost (to others, most of us), and then not to make our improvement the chief business of our lives, so that at the end of our year we go away not much better but rather worse than we came! What account can we give of such a waste of time and opportunities, of the best gifts of God, to ourselves and to Him? "For God requireth that which is past." If, when I was young, there had been such opportunities of training for Hospital work as you have, how eagerly I should have made the most of them!

Therefore, "whatsoever thy hand findeth to do, do it with all thy might" be earnest in work, be earnest also even in such things as taking exercise and proper holiday.

I say this particularly to future Matrons and Sisters, for there should be something of seriousness in keeping our bodies[7] too up to the mark.

Life is short, as preachers often tell us: that is, each stage of it is apt to come to an end before the work which belongs to it is finished. Let us

Act that each to-morrow
Find us farther than to-day.

Let us be in earnest in work: above all, because we believe this life to be the beginning of another, into which we carry with us what we have been and done here; because we are working together with God (remember the Parting Command!) and He is upholding us in our work (remember the Parting Promise!); because, when the hour of death approaches, we should wish to think (like Christ) that we have completed life, that we have finished the work which was given us to do, that we have not lost one of those, Patients or Nurses, who were entrusted to us.

What was the Parting Command?

What was the Parting Promise?

We Nurses have just kept Ascension Day and Whit-Sunday. Shall we Nurses not remember the Parting Command on Ascension Day—to preach the Gospel to every creature? And the Parting Promise: "And lo I am with you always, even unto the end of the world."

That Command and that Promise were given, not to the Apostles or Disciples only, but to each and every one of us Nurses: to each to herself in her own Ward or Home.

Without the Promise the Command could not be obeyed. Without we obey the Command the Promise will not be fulfilled.

Christ tells us what He means by the Command. He tells us, over and over again: it is by ourselves, *by what we are in ourselves*, that we are "to preach the Gospel." *Not what we say, but what we do*, is the Preacher. Not saying "Lord, Lord,"—for how many ungodly things are done and said in the name of God—but "keeping his commandments," this it is which "preaches" Him; it is the bearing much "fruit," not the saying many words. God's Spirit leads us rather to be silent than to speak, to do good works rather than to say fine things or to write them.

Over and over again, and especially in His first and last discourses, He insists upon this. He takes the sweet little child

189

and places it in our midst: it was as if He had said, "Ah! that is the best preacher of you all." And those who have followed Him best have felt this most.

The most successful preacher the world has probably seen since St. Paul's time said, some 300 years ago, it was by *showing an example*, not by delivering a discourse, that the Apostles' work was really done, that the Gospel was really preached. And well did he show his own belief in this truth. For when all was ready for his mission to convert China to Christianity, and the plague broke out where he was, he stayed and nursed the plague.

We can, every one of us here present, though our teaching may not be much, by our *lives* "preach a continual sermon, that all who see may understand." (These words were found in the last letter, left unfinished, of a native convert of the "greatest missionary of modern times," Bishop Patteson, who was martyred in the South Sea Islands, in September 1871, and this convert with him. Oh, how he puts us to shame!)

It has happened to me—I daresay it has happened to every one of us—to be told by a Child-Patient, one who had been taught to say its prayers, that it "was afraid" to kneel down and "say its prayers" before a whole ward-full of people. Do we encourage and take care of such a little child? Shall we, when we have Wards under our own charge, take care that the Ward is kept so that none at proper times shall be "afraid" to kneel down and say their prayers? Do we reflect on the immense responsibility of a Nurse towards her helpless Sick, who depend upon her almost entirely for quiet, and thought, and order? Do we think that, as was once said, we are to no one as "rude" as we are to God?

I believe that one of our St. Thomas' Sisters, who is just leaving us after years of good work, is going to set up a "Home" for Sick Children, where, under her, they will be cared for in *all* ways. I am sure that we shall all bid her "God speed." And I know that many of those who have gone out from among us, and who are now Hospital Sisters or Nurses—they would not like me to mention their names—do care for their Patients, Children and all, in *all* ways. Thank God for it!

When a Patient, especially a child, sees you acting in all things as if in the presence of God—and none are so quick to observe it—then the names he or she heard at the Chaplain's or the Sister's or the Night Nurse's lips become names of real things and real Persons. There *is* a God, a Father; there *is* a Christ, a Comforter; there *is* a Spirit of Goodness, of Holiness; there *is* another world, to such an one.

When a Patient, especially a Child, sees us acting as if there were *no* God, then there but too often becomes no God to him. Then words become to such a child mere words. And remember, that when such a Nurse—"salt" which has lost its "savour"— speaks to her Patients of God, she puts *a hindrance* in their way to keep them *from* God, instead of helping them *to* God. She had better not speak to them at all.

It is a terrible thought—I speak for myself—that we may *prevent* people from believing in God, instead of bringing them to "believe in God the Father Almighty."

What is it, "setting an example"? An example—*of what*? *Who* is *our* example, that we are to set? Christ is our example, our pattern: this we all know and say. And when this was once said—a very common word—before a very uncommon man, he said: "When you have your picture taken, the painter does not try to make it rather like, or not very unlike. It is not a good picture if it is not *exactly* like." Do we try to be *exactly* like Christ? If we do not, "are we His, or are we not?" Could it be said of each one of us: "That Nurse *is* (or is trying to be) exactly what Christ would have been in her place"?

Yet this is what every Nurse has to aim at. Aim lower: and you cannot say then, "Christ is my example." Aim as high: and, after this life, "we shall be satisfied when we awake in His likeness."

But this aim cannot be carried out, it cannot even be entertained, without the Parting Promise. The Parting Promise was fulfilled to the disciples ten days afterwards, on Whit-Sunday, when the Holy Spirit was given them—that is, when

Christ came as He promised, and was with them.

Christ comes to each Nurse of us all: and stands at our little room-door and knocks. Do we let Him in?

The Holy Spirit comes, no more with outward show but with no less inward power, to each Ward and to each Nurse of us all, who is trying to do her Nursing and her Ward work *in God*, to live her hidden Nurse's life with Christ in God.

When your Patient asks you for a drink, you do not give him a stone. And shall not our Heavenly Father much more give His Spirit to each one of us, His nurses, when she asks Him? (*Are* we *His* nurses?)

What is meant by the Spirit descending upon *us* Nurses, as it did on the first Whitsuntide? Is it not to put us in a state to nurse Him, by making our heart and our will His? (He has really told us that nursing our Patients is nursing Him.) God asks the *heart*: that is, that we should consecrate *all* our self to Him—within as well as without, *within* even more than without—in doing the Nursing work He has given each one of us here to do.

Is it not to have the spirit of love, of courtesy, of justice, of right, of gentleness, of meekness, in our Training School; the spirit of truth, of integrity, of energy and activity, of purity, which He *is*, in our Hospital? This it is to worship God in spirit and in truth. And we need not wait to go into a church, or even to kneel down at prayer, for *this* worship.

Is it not to feel that we desire really nothing for ourselves in our Nursing life, present and future, but only this, "Thy will be done," as we say in our daily prayer? Is it not to trust Him, that *His will* is really the best for each one of us? How much there is in those two words, *His will*—the will of Almighty Wisdom and Goodness, which always *knows* what is best for each one of us Nurses, which always *wills* what is best, which always *can* do what it wills for our best.

Is it not to feel that the care and thought of ourselves is lost in the thought of God and the care of our Patients and fellow-Nurses and Ward-Maids? Is it not to feel that we are never so happy as when we are working *with Him* and *for them*? And we Nurses can always do this, if we will.

Is not this what Christ meant when He said, "The kingdom of heaven is within you"? "The kingdom of heaven" consists not in much speaking but in doing, not in a sermon but in a heart. "The kingdom of heaven" can *always* be in a Nurse's blessed work, and even in her worries. Is not this what the Apostle meant when he told us to "rejoice in the Lord"? That is, to rejoice, whether Matrons, or Sisters, or Nurses, or Night Nurses, in the service of God (which, with us, means good Nursing of the Sick, good fellowship and high example as relates to our fellow-workers); to rejoice in the right, whoever does it; to rejoice in the truth, whoever has it; to rejoice in every good word and work, whoever it is; to rejoice, in one word, in what God rejoices in.

Let us thank God that some special aids to our spiritual life have been given us lately, for which I know many of us *are* thankful; and some of us have been able to keep this Whitsuntide as we never did before.

One little word more about our Training School. Training "consists in teaching people to bear responsibilities, and laying the responsibilities on them as they are able to bear them," as Bishop Patteson said of Education. The year which we spend here is generally the most important, as it may be the happiest, of our lives.

Here we find many different characters. Here we meet on a common stage, before we part company again to our several posts. If there are any rich among us, they are not esteemed for their riches. And the poor woman, the friendless, the lonely woman, receives a generous welcome.

Every one who has any activity or sense of duty may qualify herself for a future useful life. Every one may receive situations without any reference, except to individual capacity, and to a kind of capacity which it is within the power of the most humble and unfriended to work out. Every one who has any natural kindness or courtesy in her, and who is not too much wrapped up in herself, may make pleasant friends.

Although we know how many and serious faults we have, ought we not also to be able to find here some virtues which do not equally flourish in the larger world?—such as disinterested devotion to the calling we have chosen, and to which we can here fully give ourselves up without anxiety; warm-hearted interest in each other, for no one of us stands here in any other's way; freedom from jealousy and meanness; a generous self-denial in nursing our charges, and a generous sympathy with other Nurses; above all, an interest in our work, and an earnestness in taking the means given us to improve ourselves in what is to be so useful to others.

And this is also the surest sign of our improvement in it. This is what St. Paul calls: "Not slothful in business, fervent in spirit, serving the Lord."

Always, however, we must be above our work and our worries, keeping our souls free in that "hidden life" of which it has been spoken.

Above all, let us pray that God will send real workers into this immense "field" of Nursing, made more immense this year by the opening out of London *District* Nursing at the bedside of the sick poor at home. A woman who takes a sentimental view of Nursing (which she calls "ministering," as if she were an angel), is of course worse than useless. A woman possessed with the idea that she is making a sacrifice will never do; and a woman who thinks any kind of Nursing work "beneath a Nurse" will simply be in the way. But if the right woman is moved by God to come to us, what a welcome we will give her, and how happy she will soon be in a work, the many blessings of which none can know as we know them, though we know the worries too! (Good Bishop Patteson used to talk to his assistants something in this way; would we were like him!)

Nurses' work means downright work, in a cheery, happy, hopeful, friendly spirit. An earnest, bright, cheerful woman, without that notion of "making sacrifices," etc., perpetually occurring to her mind, is the real Nurse. Soldiers are sent anywhere, and leave home and country for years; *they* think nothing of it, because they go "on duty." Shall *we* have less self-denial than they, and think less of "duty" than these men? A woman with a healthy, active tone of mind, plenty of work in her, and some enthusiasm, who makes the best of everything, and, above all, does not think herself better than other people because she is a "Nightingale Nurse," that is the woman we want.

(Must I tell you again, what I have had to tell you before, that we have a great name in the world for—conceit?)

I suppose, of course, that sound religious principle is at the bottom of her.

Now, if there be any young persons really in earnest whom any of you could wish to see engaged in this work, if you know of any such, and feel justified in writing to them, you will be aiding materially in this work if you will put it in their power to propose themselves as Candidates.

My every-day thought is—"How will God provide for the introduction of real Christianity among all of us Nurses, and among our Patients?" My every-day prayer (and I know that the prayer of many of you is the same) is that He will give us the means and show us how to use them, and give us the people. We ask you to pray for us, who have to arrange for you, as we pray for you, who have to nurse the Patients; and I know you do. The very vastness of the work raises one's thoughts to God, as the only One by whom it can be done. That is the solid comfort—*He knows.* He loves us all, and our Patients infinitely more than we can. He is, we trust, sending us to them; He will bless honest endeavours to do His work among them. Without *this* belief and support, it seems to me, when we look at the greatness of the work, and how far, far we fall short of it, instead of being conceited, we should not have courage to work at all.

And when we say the words in the Communion Service—"Therefore with angels and archangels," do we think whether we are fit company for angels? It may not be fanciful to believe that "angels and archangels," to whom all must seem so different, may see God's light breaking over the Nursing Service, though perhaps in our time it may not attain the perfect day. Only we must work on, and bring no hindrances to that light. And that not one of us may bring hindrances to that light, believe me, let us pray daily.

I have been longer than I intended or hoped, and will only say one more word.

May we each and all of us Nurses be faithful to the end, remembering this, that no one Nurse stands alone. May we not say, in the words of the prophet, that it is "The Lord" who "hath gathered" us Nurses "together out of the lands"? "It is because we do not *praise* as we proceed," said a good and great man, "that our progress is so slow." Should not all this Training School be so melted into one heart and mind, that we may with *one* heart and mind act and nurse and sing together our praise and thanksgiving, blessing and gratitude, for mercies, every one of which seems to belong to the whole School? For every Nurse alike belongs to the Mother School of which she is a part, and to the Almighty Father, who has sent her here, and to whom alone we each and all of us Nurses owe everything we have and are.

F. N.

V

April 28, 1876.

My dear Friends,—Again another year has brought us together to rejoice at our successes, and, if to grieve over some disappointments, to try together to find out what it is that may have brought them about, and to correct it.

God seems to have given His favour to the manner in which you have been working.

Thanks to you, each and all of you, for the pains you have taken to carry out the work. I hope you feel how great have been the pains bestowed upon you.

You are not "grumblers" at all: you do try to justify the great care given you, the confidence placed in you, and, after you have left this Home, the freedom of action you enjoy—by that *intelligent* obedience to rules and orders, to render which is alone worthy of the name of "Trained Nurse," of God's soldier. We shall be poor soldiers indeed, if we don't *train* ourselves for the battle. But if discipline is ever looked upon as interference, then freedom has become lawlessness, and we are no "Trained Nurses" at all.

The trained Englishwoman is the first Nurse in the world: *if*—IF she knows how to unite this intelligent obedience to commands with thoughtful and godly command of herself.

"The greatest evils in life," said one of the world's highest statesmen, "have had their rise from something which was thought of too little importance to attend to." How we Nurses can echo that!

"Immense, incalculable misery" is due to "the immoral thoughtlessness"—he calls thoughtlessness immoral—of women about little things. This is what our training is to counteract in us. Think nothing too small to be attended to in this way. Think everything too small of personal trouble or sensitiveness to be cared for in another way.

It is not knowledge only: it is practice we want. We only *know* a thing if we can *do* it. There is a famous Italian proverb which says: "So much"—and no more—"each knows as she does."

What we did last year we may look upon not as a matter of conceit, but of encouragement. We must not fail this year, and we'll not fail. We'll keep up to the mark: nay more, we will press on to a higher mark. For our "calling" is a high one (the "little things," remember: a high excellence in little things). And we must answer to the call ever more and more strenuously and ever more and more humbly too.

We live together: let us live for each other's comfort. We are all working together: grasp the idea of this as a larger work than our own little pet hobbies, which are very narrow, our own little personal wishes, feelings, piques, or tempers. This is not individual work. A real Nurse sinks self. Remember we are not so many small selves, but members of a community.

"Little children, love one another." To love, that is, to help one another, to strive together, to act together, to work for the same end, to bring to perfection the sisterly feeling of fellow-workers, without which nothing great is done, nothing good lasts. Might not St. John have been thinking of us Nurses in our Training Schools when he said that?

May God be with us all and we be *one* in Him and in His *work*!

God speed us all!
Amen in our hearts.

These are some of the little things we need to attend to:

To be a Nurse *is* to be a Nurse: not to be a Nurse only when we are put to the work we like. If we can't work when we are put to the work we don't like—and Patients can't always be fitted to Nurses—that is behaving like a spoilt child, like a naughty girl: not like a Nurse.

If we can do the work we don't like from the higher motive till we do like it, that is one test of being a real Nurse. A Nurse is not one who can only do what she does like, and can't do what she does not like. For the Patients want according to their wants, and not according to the Nurse's likes or dislikes.

If you wish to be trained to do *all* Nursing well, even what you do not like—trained to perfection in little things—that is Nursing for the sake of Nursing, for the sake of God and of your neighbour. And remember, in little things as in great—No Cross, no Crown.

Nursing is said, most truly said, to be a high calling, an honourable calling.

But what does the honour lie in? In working hard during your training to learn and to do all things perfectly. The honour does not lie in putting on Nursing like your uniform, your dress; though dishonour often lies in being neat in your uniform within doors and dressy in your finery out of doors. Dishonour always lies in inconsistency.

Honour lies in loving perfection, consistency, and in working hard for it: in being ready to work patiently: ready to say not "How clever I am!" but "I am not yet worthy: but Nursing is worthy; and I will live to deserve and work to deserve to be called a Trained Nurse."

Here are two of the plain, practical, little things necessary to produce good Nurses, the want of attention to which produces some of the "greatest evils in life": quietness, cleanliness, (*a*) Quietness in moving about the "Home"; in arranging your rooms, in not *slamming* every door after you. No noisy talking on the stairs and in the lobbies—forgetting at times some unfortunate Night Nurse in bed. But if you are Nurses, Nurses ought to be going about quietly whether Night Nurses are asleep or not. For a Sick Ward ought to be as quiet as a Sick Room; and a Sick Room, I need not say, ought to be the quietest place in God's Kingdom. Quietness in dress, especially being *consistent* in this matter when off duty and going out. And oh! let the Lady Probationers realise how important their example is in these things, so little and so great! If you are Nurses, Nurses ought not to be dressy, whether in or out of their uniform.

Do you remember that Christ holds up the wild flowers as our example in dress? Why? He says: God "clothes" the field flowers. How does He clothe them?

First: their "clothes" are exactly suitable for the kind of place they are in and the kind of work they have to do. So should ours be.

Second: field flowers are never double: double flowers change their useful stamens for showy petals, and so have no seeds. These double flowers are like the useless appendages now worn on the dress, and very much in your way. Wild flowers have purpose in all their beauty. So ought dress to have; nothing purposeless about it.

Third: the colours of the wild flower are perfect in harmony, and not many of them.

Fourth: there is not a speck on the freshness with which flowers come out of the dirty earth. Even when our clothes are getting rather old we may imitate the flower: for we may make them look as fresh as a daisy.

Whatsoever we do, whether we eat or drink *or dress*, let us do all to the glory of God. But above all remember, "Be not anxious what ye shall put on," which is the real meaning of "Take no thought."

This is not my own idea: it was in a Bible lesson, never to be forgotten. And I knew a Nurse who dressed so nicely and quietly after she had heard this Bible lesson that you would think of her as a model. And alas! I have known, oh how many! whose dress was their snare.

Oh, my dear Nurses, whether gentlewomen or not, don't let people say of you that you are like "Girls of the Period": let them say that you are like "field flowers," and welcome.

(*b*) Cleanliness in person and in our rooms, thinking nothing too small to be attended to in this respect. And if these things are important in the "Home," think how important they are in the

Wards, where cleanliness and fresh air—there can be no pure air without cleanliness—not so much give life as *are* the very life of the Patients; where the smallest carelessness may turn the scale from life to death; where Disinfectants, as one of your own Surgeons has said, are but a "mystic rite." Cleanliness is the only real Disinfectant. Remember that Typhoid Fever is distinctly a filth disease; that Consumption is distinctly the product of breathing foul air, especially at night; that in surgical cases, Erysipelas and Pyaemia are simply a poisoning of the blood—generally thro' some want of cleanliness or other. And do not speak of these as little things, which determine the most momentous issues of life and death. I knew a Probationer who when washing a poor man's ulcerated leg, actually wiped it on his sheet, and excused herself by saying she had always seen it done so in another place. The least carelessness in not washing your hands between one bad case and another, and many another carelessness which it is plain I cannot mention here—it would not be nice, though it is much less nice to do it—the least carelessness, I say, in these things which every Nurse can be careful or careless in, may cost a life: aye, may cost your own, or at least a finger. We have all seen poisoned fingers.

I read with more interest than if they were novels your case papers. Some are meagre, especially in the "history." Some are good. Please remember that, besides your own instruction, you can give me some too, by making these most interesting cases as interesting as possible, by making them full and accurate, and entering the full history. If the history of every case were recorded, especially of Typhoid Fever, which is, as we said, a filth disease, it is impossible to over-estimate the body of valuable information which would thus be got together, and might go far, in the hands of Officers of Health and by recent laws, to prevent disease altogether. The District Nurses are most useful in this respect.

When we obey all God's laws as to cleanliness, fresh air, pure water, good habits, good dwellings, good drains, food and drink, work and exercise, health is the result. When we disobey, sickness. 110,000 lives are needlessly sacrificed every year in this kingdom by our disobedience, and 220,000 people are needlessly sick all the year round. And why? Because we will not know, will not obey God's simple Health laws.

No epidemic can resist thorough cleanliness and fresh air.

Is there any Nurse here who is a Pharisee? This seems a very cruel and unjust question.

We think of the Pharisees, when we read the terrible denunciation of them by our Master, as a small, peculiar, antiquated sect of 2000 years ago. Are they not rather the least peculiar, the most widely-spread people of every time? I am sure I often ask myself, sadly enough, "Am I a Pharisee?" In this sense: Am I, or am I not, doing this with a single eye to God's work, to serving Him and my neighbour, even tho' my "neighbour" is as hostile to me as the Jew was to the Samaritan? Or am I doing it because I identify my selfish self with the work, and in so doing serve myself and not God? If so, then I am a Pharisee.

It is good to love our Training School and our body, and to wish to keep up its credit. We are bound to do so. That is helping God's work in the world. We are bound to try to be the "salt of the world" in nursing; but if we are conceited, seeking *ourselves* in this, then we are not "salt" but Pharisees.

We should have zeal for God's sake and His work's sake: but some seem to have zeal for zeal's sake only. Zeal does not make a Christian Nurse if it is zeal for our own credit and glory—tho' Christ was the most zealous mediciner that ever was. (He says: "The zeal of God's house hath eaten me up.") Zeal by itself does not make a good Nurse: it makes a Pharisee. Christ is so strong upon this point of not being conceited, of not nursing to show what "fine fellows" we are as Nurses, that He actually says "it is conceited of us to let one of our hands know what the other does." What will He say if He sees one of us doing all her work to let not only her other hand but other people know she does it? Yet all our best work which looks so well *may* be done from this motive.

And let me tell you a little secret. One of our Superintendents at a distance says that she finds she must not boast so much about St. Thomas'. Nor must you. People have heard too much about it. I dare say you remember the fine old Greek statesman who was banished because people were tired of hearing him called "The Just." Don't let people get tired of hearing you call St. Thomas' "The Just" when you are away from us. We shall not at all complain of your proving it "The Just" by your training and conduct.

I read lately in a well-known medical journal, speaking of the "Nightingale Nurses," that the day is quite gone by when a novel would give a caricature of a Nurse as a "Mrs. Gamp"—drinking, brutal, ignorant, coarse old woman. The "Nightingale Nurse" in a novel, it said, would be—what do you think?—an active, useful, clever Nurse. These are the parts I approve of. But what else do you think?—a lively, rather pert, and very conceited young woman. Ah, there's the rub. You see what our name is "up" for in the world. That's what I should like to be left out. This is what a friendly critic says of us, and we may be very sure that unfriendly critics say much worse. Do we deserve what they say of us? That is the question. Let us not have, each one of us, to say "yes" in our own hearts. Christ made no light matter of conceit.

Keep the usefulness, and let the conceit go.

And may I here say a few words of counsel to those who may be called upon to be Night Nurses? One of these asked me with tears to pray for her. I do pray for all of you, our dear Night Nurses. In my restless nights my thoughts turn to you incessantly by the bedsides of restless and suffering Patients, and I pray God that He will make, thro' you, thro' your patience, your skill, your hope, faith and charity, every Ward into a Church, and teach us that to *be* the Gospel is the only way to "preach the Gospel," which Christ tells us is the duty of every one of us "unto the end of the world"—every woman and Nurse of us all; and that a collection of any people trying to live like Christ is a Church.

Did you ever think how Christ was a Nurse, and stood by the bed, and with His own hands nursed and "did for" the sufferers?

But, to return to those who may be called upon to be Night Nurses: do not abuse the liberty given you on emerging from the "Home," where you are cared for as if you were our children. Keep to regular hours by day for your meals, your sleep, your exercise. If you do not, you will never be able to do and stand the night work perfectly; if you do, there is no reason why night nursing may not be as healthy as day. (I used to be very fond of the night when I was a Night Nurse; I know what it is. But then I had my day work to do besides; you have not.) Do not turn dressy in your goings out by day. It is vulgar, it is mean, to burst out into freedom in this way. There are circumstances of peculiar temptation when, after the restraint and motherly care of the "Home," you, the young ones, are put into circumstances of peculiar liberty. Is it not the time to act like Daniel?... Let "the Judge, the Righteous Judge," have to call us not the "Pharisees," but Daniel's band!

That is what I pray for you, for me, for all of us.

But what is it to be a Daniel's band? What is God's command to Night Nurses? It is—is it not?—not to slur over any duty—not the very least of all our duties—as Night Nurse: to be able to give a full, accurate, and minute account of each Patient the next morning: to be strictly reserved in your manner with gentlemen ("Thou God seest me": no one else); to be honest and true. You don't know how well the Patients know you, how accurately they judge you. You can do them no good unless they see that you *live* what you say.

It is: not to go out showily dressed, and not to keep irregular hours with others in the day time.

> Dare to have a purpose firm,
> Dare to make it known.

Watch—watch. Christ seems to have had a special word for

Night Nurses: "I say unto you, watch." And He says: "Lo, I am with you alway," when no one else is by.

And he divides us all, at this moment, into the "wise virgins" and the "foolish virgins." Oh, let Him not find any "foolish virgins" among our Night Nurses! Each Night Nurse has to stand alone in her Ward.

Dare to stand alone.

Let our Master be able to say some day that every one of the Patients has been the better, not only in body but in spirit—whether going to life or to death—for having been nursed by each one of you.

But one is gone, perhaps the dearest of all—Nurse Martha Rice.

I was the last to see her in England. She was so pleased to be going to Miss Machin at Montreal. She said it was no sacrifice, except the leaving her parents. She almost wished it had been, that she might have had something to give to God.

Now she *has* had something to give to God: her life.

"So young, so happy: all so happy together, when in their room they were always sitting round the table, so cheerful, reading their Bible together. She walked round the garden so happy that last night."

So pure and fresh: there was something of the sweet savour of holiness about her. I could tell you of souls upon whom she made a great impression: all unknowing: simply by being herself.

A noble sort of girl: sound and holy in mind and heart: living with God. It is scarcely respectful to say how I liked her, now she is an angel in heaven; like a child to Miss Machin, who was like a mother to her, loved and nursed her day and night.

"So dear and bright a creature," "liked and respected by every one in the Hospital," "and, as a Nurse, hardly too much can be said in her favour." "To the Doctors, Patients, and Superintendent, she was simply invaluable." "The contrast between these Nurses and the best of others is to be keenly felt daily"; "doing bravely"; "perfectly obedient and pleasant to their Superintendent."

Was Martha conceited with all this? She was one of the simplest humblest Christian women I have ever known. All noble souls are simple, natural, and humble.

Let us be like her, and, like her, not conceited with it all. She was too brave to be conceited: too brave not to be humble. *She* had trained herself for the battle.

"With a nice, genial, respectful manner, which never left her, great firmness in duty, and steadiness that rendered her above suspicion": "happy and interested in her charge."

More above all petty calculations about self, all paltry wranglings, than almost any. How different for us, for her, had it not been so! Could we have mourned her as we do? The others of the small Montreal staff who miss her so terribly will like to hear how we feel this. They were all with her when she died. Miss Machin sat up with her every night, and either she or Miss Blower never left her, day or night, during the last nine days of her illness. She died of typhoid fever: peritonitis the last three weeks; but, as she had survived so long, they hoped against hope up to Easter Day.

About seven days before her death, during her delirium, she said: "The Lord has two wills: His will be done." It is when we do not know what God's will is to be, that it is the hardest to will what He wills.

Strange to say, on Good Friday, though she was so delirious that there was difficulty in keeping her in bed, and she did not know what day it was, Christ on the Cross was her theme all the day long. "Christ died on the Cross for me, and I want to go and die for Him." She had indeed lived for Him. Then on Easter Day she said to Miss Blower: "I am happy, so happy: we are both happy, so very happy." She said she was going to hear the eighth Psalm. Shall we remember Martha's favourite psalm? She spoke often about St. Thomas'.

She died the day after Easter Day. The change came at 7 in the evening, and she lived till 5 o'clock the next morning, conscious to the last, repeating sentences, and answering by looks when she could speak no more. Her Saviour, whom she had so loved and followed in her life, was with her thro' the Valley of the Shadow of Death, and she felt Him there. She was happy. "My best love," she said, "tell them it is all for the best, and I am not sorry I came out."

Her parents have given her up nobly, though with bleeding hearts, with true submission to our Father's will: they *are* satisfied it is "all for the best."

All the Montreal Hospital shared our sorrow. The Doctors were full of kindness in their medical attendance. Mr. Redpath, who is a principal Director, and Mrs. Redpath were like a real father and mother to our people. Martha's death-bed and coffin were strewed with flowers.

Public and private prayers were offered up for her at Montreal during her illness. Who can say that they were not answered?

She spoke of dying: but without fear. We prayed that God would spare the child to us: but He had need of her.

Our Father arranged her going out: for she went, if ever woman did, with a single eye to please Him and do her duty to the work and her Superintendent. "Is it well with the child?" "It is well." Let us who feel her loss so deeply in the work not grudge her to God.

As one of you yourselves said: "She died like a good soldier of Jesus Christ, well to the front." Would any one of us wish it otherwise for her? Would any one of us wish a better lot for herself? There is but one feeling among us all about her: that she lived as a noble Christian girl, and that she has been permitted to die nobly: in the post of honour, as a soldier thinks it glorious to die. In the midst of our work, so surely do we Nurses think it glorious to die.

But to be like her we must have a mind like hers: "enduring, patient, firm, and meek." I know that she sought of God the mind of Jesus Christ, "active, like His; like His, resigned"; copying His pattern: ready to "endure hardness."

We give her joy; it is our loss, not hers. She is gone to our Lord and her Lord, made ripe so soon for her and our Father's house. Our tears are her joy. She is in another room of our Father's house. She bids us now give thanks for her. Think of that Easter morn when she rose again! She had indeed "another morn than ours"—that 17th of April.

FLORENCE NIGHTINGALE.

VI

Easter Eve, 1879, 6 A.M.

My dear Friends,—I am always thinking of you, and as my Easter greeting, I could not help copying for you part of a letter which one of my brother-in-law's family had from Col. Degacher (commanding one battalion of the 24th Regiment in Natal), giving the names of men whom he recommended for the Victoria Cross, when defending the Commissariat Stores at Rorke's Drift. (His brother, Capt. Degacher, was killed at Isandhlwana.) He says:

"Private John Williams was posted, together with Private Joseph Williams and Private William Harrison (1/24th Regiment), in a further ward of the Hospital. They held it for more than an hour—so long as they had a round of ammunition left, when, as communication was for the time cut off, the Zulus were enabled to advance and burst open the door. A hand-to-hand conflict then ensued, during which Private Joseph Williams and two of the Patients were dragged out and assegaied (killed with a short spear or dagger).

"Whilst the Zulus were occupied with the slaughter of these

unfortunate men, a lull took place, which enabled Private John Williams (who with two of the Patients were by this time the *only men left alive* in the Ward) to succeed in knocking a hole in the partition and taking the two Patients with him into the next ward, where he found Private Henry Hook.

"These two men together, one man working whilst the other fought and held the enemy at bay with his bayonet, broke through three more partitions, and were thus enabled to bring eight Patients through a small window into the inner line of defence.

"In another ward facing the hill, William Jones and Private Robert Jones had been placed: they defended their post to the last, and until six out of seven Patients it contained had been removed. The seventh, Sergeant Maxfield, 2/24th Regiment, was delirious from fever, and although they had previously dressed him, they were unable to induce him to move; and when Private Robert Jones returned to endeavour to carry him off, he found him being stabbed on his bed by the Zulus.

"Corporal Wm. Allen and Fd. Hitch, 2/24th Regiment, must also be mentioned. It was chiefly due to their courageous conduct that communication with the Hospital was kept up at all—holding together, at all costs, a most dangerous post, raked in reverse by the enemy's fire from the hill. They were both severely wounded, but their determined conduct enabled the Patients to be withdrawn from the Hospital. And when incapacitated from their wounds from fighting themselves, they continued, as soon as their wounds were dressed, to serve out ammunition to their comrades throughout the night."

These men who were defending the house at Rorke's Drift were 120 of his (Col. Degacher's) men against 5000 Zulus, and they fought from 3 P.M. of January 22nd, to 5 A.M. of the 23rd. *There* is a Night Nurse's work for you. "When shall such heroes live again?" In every Nurse of us all. Every Nurse may at all costs serve her Patients as these brave heroic men did at the risk and the cost of their own lives.

Three cheers for these bravest of Night Nurses of Rorke's Drift, who regarded not themselves, not their ease, not even their lives; who regarded duty and discipline; who stood to the last by God and their neighbour; who saved their post and their Patients. And may we Nurses all be like them, and fight through the night for our Patients' lives—fight through every night and day!

Do you see what a high feeling of comradeship does for these men? Many a soldier loses his life in the field by going back to help a drowning or a wounded comrade, who might have saved it. Oh, let us Nurses all be *comrades*; stick to the honour of our flag and our corps, and help each other to the best success, for the sake of Him who died, as at this time, to save us all!

And let us remember that petty selfishnesses and meannesses and self-indulgences hinder our honour as good soldiers of Jesus Christ and of the Unseen God, who sees all these little things when no one else does!

What makes us endure to the end? Discipline. Do you think these men could thus have fought at a desperate post through the livelong night if they had not been trained to obedience to orders, and to acting as a corps, yet each man doing his own duty to the fullest extent—rather than every man going his own way, thinking of his own likings, and caring for himself?

How *great* may be men and women, "little lower than the angels," and also how *little*!

Humility—to think our own life worth nothing except as serving in a corps, God's nursing corps, unflinching obedience, steadiness, and endurance in carrying out His work—that is true discipline, that is true greatness, and may God give it to us Nurses, and make us His own Nurses.

And let us not think that these things can be done in a day or a night. No, they are the result of no rough-and-ready method. The most important part of those efforts was to be found in the patient labour of years. These great tasks are not to be accomplished suddenly by raw fellows in a night; it is when discipline and training have become a kind of second nature to us that they can be accomplished every day and every night. The raw Native levies ran away, determining our fall at Isandhlwana. The well-trained English soldiers, led by their Officers and their Non-commissioned Officers, stuck to their posts.

Every feeling, every thought we have, stamps a character upon us, especially in our year of training, and in the next year or two.

The most unruly boys, weak in themselves—for unruliness is weakness—when they have to submit, it brings out all the good points in their characters. These boys, so easily led astray, they put themselves under the severest discipline, and after training sometimes come out the best of us all. The qualities which, when let alone, run to seed and do themselves and others nothing but harm, under proper discipline make fine fellows of them.

And what is it to obey? To obey means to do what we are told, and to do it at once. With the nurse, as with the soldier, whether we have been accustomed to it or not, whether we think it right or not, is not the question. Prompt obedience is the question. We are not in control, but under control. Prompt obedience is the first thing; the rest is traditional nonsense. But mind who we go to for our orders. Go to headquarters. True discipline is to uphold authority, and not to mind trouble. We come into the work to do the work....

We Nurses are taught the "reason why," as soldiers cannot be, of much of what we have to do. But it would be making a poor use of this "reason why" if we were to turn round in any part of our training and say, or *not* say, but *feel*—We know better than you.

Would we be of less use than the Elephant? The Elephant who could kill a hundred men, but who alike pushes the artillery train with his head when the horses cannot move it, and who minds the children and carefully nurses them, and who threads a needle with his trunk. Why? Because he has been taught to *obey*. He would be of no use but to destroy, unless he had learnt that. Sometimes he has a strong will, and it is not easy for him to get his lesson perfect. We can feel for him. We know a little about it ourselves. But he does learn in time to go our way and not his own, to carry a heavy load, which of course he would rather not do, to turn to which ever side we wish, and to stop when we want him to stop.

So God teaches each one of us in time to go His way and not our own. And one of the best things I can wish each one of us is that we may learn the Elephant's lesson, that is to obey, in good time and not too late.

Pray for me, my dear friends, that I may learn it, even in my old age.

FLORENCE NIGHTINGALE.

VII

London, *May 16, 1888.*

My dear Friends,—Here, one year more, is my very best love and heart-felt "good speed" to the work.

To each and to all I wish the very highest success, in the widest meaning of the word, in the life's work you have chosen.

And I am more sorry than for anything else that my illness, more than usually serious, has let me know personally so little of you, except through our dear Matron and dear Home Sister.

You are going steadily and devotedly on in preparing yourselves for future work. Accept my heartiest sympathy and thanks.

We hear much of "Associations" now. It is impossible indeed to live in isolation: we are dependent upon others for the supply of all our wants, and others upon us.

Every Hospital is an "Association" in itself. *We* of this School are an Association in the deepest sense, regulated—at least we strive towards it—on high and generous principles; through organisation working at once for our own and our fellow Nurses' success. For, to make progress possible, we must make this interdependence a source of good: not a means of standing still.

There is no magic in the word "Association," but there is a secret, a mighty call in it, *if* we will but listen to the "still small voice" in it, calling upon each of us to do our best.

It calls upon our dear heads, and they answer. It calls upon each of us.

We must never forget that the "Individual" makes the Association. What the Association *is* depends upon each of its members. A Nurses' Association can never be a substitute for the individual Nurse. It is she who must, each in her measure, give life to the Association, while the Association helps *her*.

We *have* our dear heads. Thank God for them! Let us each one of us be a living member, according to her several ability. It is the individual that signifies—rather than the law or the rule.

Has not every one who has experience of the world been struck by this: you may have the most admirable circumstances and organisations and examinations and certificates, yet, if the individual allows herself to sink to a lower level, it is all but a "tinkling cymbal" for her. It is how the circumstances are worked that signifies. Circumstances are opportunities.

Rules may become a dead letter. It is the spirit of them that "giveth life." It is the individual, inside, that counts, the level she is upon which tells. The rest is only the outward shell or envelope. She must become a "rule of thought" to herself through the Ruler.

And on the other hand, it strikes you often, as a great man has said, if the individual finds herself afterwards in less admirable circumstances, but keeps her high level, and rises to a higher and a higher level still—if she makes of her difficulties, her opportunities—steps to ascend—she commands her circumstances; she is capable of the best Nursing work and spirit, capable of the best influence over her Patients.

It is again, what the individual Nurse *is* and can do during her *living* training and *living* work that signifies, not what she is certified for, like a steam-boiler, which is certified to stand so much pressure of work.

She may have gone through a first-rate course, plenty of examinations, and we may find nothing inside. It may be the difference between a Nurse nursing, and a Nurse reading a book on Nursing. Unless it bear fruit, it is all gilding and veneering: the reality is not there, growing, growing every year. Every Nurse must grow. No Nurse can stand still. She must go forward or she will go backward every year.

And how can a Certificate or public Register show this? Rather, she ought to have a moral "Clinical" Thermometer in herself. Our stature does not grow every year after we are "grown up." Neither does it grow down. It is otherwise with our moral stature and our Nursing stature. We grow down, if we don't grow up, every year.

At the present time, when there are so many Associations, when periodicals and publicity are so much the fashion, when there is such a dragging of everything before the public, there is some danger of our forgetting that any true Nursing work must be quiet work—an individual work. Anything else is contrary to the whole realness of the work. *Where* am *I*, the individual, in my inmost soul? *What* am *I*, the inner woman called "I"? That is the question.

This "I" must be quiet yet quick; quick without hurry; gentle without slowness, discreet without self-importance. "In quietness and in confidence must be her strength."

I must be trustworthy, to carry out directions intelligently and perfectly, *unseen* as well as seen; "unto the Lord" *as well as* unto men; no mere eye service. (How can this be if she is a mere Association Nurse, and not an individual Nurse?)

I must have moral influence over my Patients. And I *can* only have this by *being* what I appear, especially now that everybody is educated, so that Patients become my keen critics and judges. My Patients are watching me. They know what my profession, my calling is: to devote myself to the good of the sick. They are asking themselves: does that Nurse act up to her profession? This is no supposition. It is a fact. It is a call to us, to each individual Nurse, to act up to her profession.

We hear a good deal nowadays about Nursing being made a "profession." Rather, is it not the question for *me*: *am I* living up to my "profession"?

But I must not crave for the Patient to be always recognising my services. On the contrary: the best service I can give is that the Patient shall scarcely be aware of any—shall recognise my presence most by recognising that he has *no* wants.

Shakespeare tells me that to be "nurse like" is to be to the Patient—

So kind, so duteous, diligent,
So tender over his occasions, true,
So feat.

I must be thorough—a work, not a word—a Nurse, not a book, not an answer, not a certificate, not a mechanism, a mere piece of a mechanism or Association.

At the same time, in as far as Associations really give help and pledges for progress, are not mere crutches, stereotypes for standing still, let us bid them "God speed" with our whole hearts.

We all know what "parasites" are, plants or animals which live upon others and don't work for their own food, and so degenerate. For the work to get food is quite as necessary as the food itself for healthy active life and development.

Now, there is a danger in the air of becoming Parasites in Nursing (and also Midwifery)—of our becoming Nurses (and Midwives) by deputy, a danger now when there is so great an inclination to make school and college education, all sorts of Sciences and Arts, even Nursing and Midwifery, a book and examination business, a profession in the low, not in the high sense of the word. And the danger is that we shall be content to let the book and the theory and the words do for us. One of the most religious of men says that we let the going to Church and the clergyman do for us *instead of* the learning and the practice, if we have the Parasite tendency, and that even the better the service and the better the sermon and the theory and the teaching, the more danger there is that we may let it do. He says that we may become satisfied to be prayed for instead of praying—to have our work for Christ done by a paid deputy—to be fed by a deputy who gives us our supply for a week—to substitute for thought what is meant as a stimulus to thought and practice. This is the parasite of the pew he says (as the literary parasite thinks he knows everything because he has a "good library"). He enjoys his weekly, perhaps his daily worship, while character and life, will and practice are not only not making progress, but are actually deteriorating.

Do you remember Tennyson's farmer, who says of the clergyman:

> I 'eärd 'um a bummin' awaäy ... ower my 'eäd, . . .
> An' I thowt a said whot a owt to 'a said an' I coom'd awaäy.

We laugh at that. But is the Parasite much better than that?

Now the Ambulance Classes, the Registration, the Certificates of Nursing and of Nurses (and of midwifery), especially any which may demand the minimum of *practice*, which may *substitute* for *personal* progress in active proficiency, mere literary or word progress, instead of making it the material for growth in correct knowledge and practice, all such like things may tend this way.

It is not the certificate which makes the Nurse or the Midwife. It may *un-make* her. The danger is lest she let the certificate be *instead of* herself, *instead of* her own never ceasing going up higher as a woman and a Nurse.

This is the "day" of Examinations in the turn that Education—

Elementary, the Higher Education, Professional Education—seems taking. And it is a great step which has substituted this for what used to be called "interest." Only let us never allow it to encroach upon what cannot be tested by examinations. Only let the "day" of *Practice*, the development of each individual's thought and practice, character and dutifulness, keep up, through the materials given us for growth and for correct knowledge, with the "day of examinations" in the Nurse's life, which is above all a moral and practical life, a life not of show, but of faithful action.

But above all, dear comrades, let each one of us, each individual of us, not only bid "God speed" in her heart to this, our own School (or Association—call it so if you will), but *strive* to *speed* it with all the best that is in her, even as your "Association" and its dear heads strive to speed each one of you.

Let each one of us take the abundant and excellent food for the mind which is offered us, in our training, our classes, our lectures, our examinations and reading—not as "Parasites," no, none of you will ever do that—but as bright and vigorous fellow-workers, working out the better way every day to the end of life.

Once more, my heartiest sympathy, my dearest love to each and to all of you, from your ever faithful old comrade,

Florence Nightingale.

FOOTNOTES:

[1] The beginning of the first address will suggest a reason for this turn of phrase. A nurse who had been through training might not always be "worthy of the name of 'Trained Nurse' " (Address of 1876).

[2] There is a well-known Society abroad (for charitable works) of which the Members go through a two years' probation on their first entering, but after ten years they return and go through a second probation of one year. This is one of the most striking recognitions I know of the fact that progress is always to be made: that grown-up people, even of middle-age, ought always to have their education going on. But only those *can* learn *after* middle age who have gone on learning up to middle age.

[3] The Madre Santa Colomba, of the Convent of the Trinità dei Monti in Rome.—Editor's Note.

[4] There is a most suggestive story told of one, some 300 years ago, an able and learned man, who presented himself for admission into a Society for Preaching and Charitable Works. He was kept for many months on this query: *Are you a Christian?* by his "Master of Probationers." He took kindly and heartily to it; went with his whole soul and mind into this little momentous question, and solved it victoriously in his own course, and in his after course of usefulness for others. Am I a Christian? is most certainly the first and most important question for each one of us Nurses. Let us ask it, each of herself, every day.

[5] Nightingale Nurse and Lady Superintendent of Liverpool Workhouse Infirmary. Pioneer of Workhouse Nursing. After her early death in 1868 Miss Nightingale wrote in *Good Words* an article, "Una and the Lion," on her life and work.—Editor's Note.

[6] Madame Caroline Werckner, an Englishwoman.—Editor's Note.

[7] Do you remember the word of one of the greatest poets of the Middle Ages?

218

NURSING —
WHAT IT IS, AND
WHAT IT IS NOT.

By Florence Nightingale, 1860

DISEASE A REPARATIVE PROCESS.

Shall we begin by taking it as a general principle—that all disease, at some period or other of its course, is more or less a reparative process, not necessarily accompanied with suffering: an effort of nature to remedy a process of poisoning or of decay, which has taken place weeks, months, sometimes years beforehand, unnoticed, the termination of the disease being then, while the antecedent process was going on, determined?

If we accept this as a general principle we shall be immediately met with anecdotes and instances to prove the contrary. Just so if we were to take, as a principle—all the climates of the earth are meant to be made habitable for man, by the efforts of man—the objection would be immediately raised,—Will the top of Mont Blanc ever be made habitable? Our answer would be, it will be many thousands of years before we have reached the bottom of Mont Blanc in making the earth healthy. Wait till we have reached the bottom before we discuss the top.

OF THE SUFFERINGS OF DISEASE,
DISEASE NOT ALWAYS THE CAUSE.

In watching disease, both in private houses and in public hospitals, the thing which strikes the experienced observer most forcibly is this, that the symptoms or the sufferings generally considered to be inevitable and incident to the disease are very often not symptoms of the disease at all, but of something quite different—of the want of fresh air, or of light, or of warmth, or of quiet, or of cleanliness, or of punctuality and care in the administration of diet, of each or of all of these. And this quite as much in private as in hospital nursing.

The reparative process which Nature has instituted and which we call disease has been hindered by some want of knowledge or attention, in one or in all of these things, and pain, suffering, or interruption of the whole process sets in.

If a patient is cold, if a patient is feverish, if a patient is faint, if he is sick after taking food, if he has a bed-sore, it is generally the fault not of the disease, but of the nursing.

WHAT NURSING OUGHT TO DO.

I use the word nursing for want of a better. It has been limited to signify little more than the administration of medicines and the application of poultices. It ought to signify the proper use of fresh air, light, warmth, cleanliness, quiet, and the proper selection and administration of diet—all at the least expense of vital power to the patient.

NURSING THE SICK LITTLE UNDERSTOOD.

It has been said and written scores of times, that every woman makes a good nurse. I believe, on the contrary, that the very elements of nursing are all but unknown.

By this I do not mean that the nurse is always to blame. Bad sanitary, bad architectural, and bad administrative arrangements often make it impossible to nurse.

But the art of nursing ought to include such arrangements as alone make what I understand by nursing, possible.

The art of nursing, as now practised, seems to be expressly constituted to unmake what God had made disease to be, viz., a reparative process.

NURSING OUGHT TO
ASSIST THE REPARATIVE PROCESS.

To recur to the first objection. If we are asked, Is such or such a disease a reparative process? Can such an illness be unaccompanied with suffering? Will any care prevent such a patient from suffering this or that?—I humbly say, I do not know. But when you have done away with all that pain and suffering, which in patients are the symptoms not of their disease, but of the absence of one or all of the above-mentioned essentials to the success of Nature's reparative processes, we shall then know what are the symptoms of and the sufferings inseparable from the disease.

Another and the commonest exclamation which will be instantly made is—Would you do nothing, then, in cholera, fever, &c.?—so deep-rooted and universal is the conviction that to give medicine is to be doing something, or rather everything; to give air, warmth, cleanliness, &c., is to do nothing. The reply is, that in these and many other similar diseases the exact value of particular remedies and modes of treatment is by no means ascertained, while there is universal experience as to the extreme importance of careful nursing in determining the issue of the disease.

NURSING THE WELL.

II. The very elements of what constitutes good nursing are as little understood for the well as for the sick. The same laws of health or of nursing, for they are in reality the same, obtain among the well as among the sick. The breaking of them produces only a less violent consequence among the former than among the latter,—and this sometimes, not always.

It is constantly objected,—"But how can I obtain this medical knowledge? I am not a doctor. I must leave this to doctors."

LITTLE UNDERSTOOD.

Oh, mothers of families! You who say this, do you know that one in every seven infants in this civilized land of England perishes before it is one year old? That, in London, two in every five die before they are five years old? And, in the other great cities of England, nearly one out of two?[1] "The life duration of tender babies" (as some Saturn, turned analytical chemist, says) "is the most delicate test" of sanitary conditions. Is all this premature suffering and death necessary? Or did Nature intend mothers to be always accompanied by doctors? Or is it better to learn the piano-forte than to learn the laws which subserve the preservation of offspring?

Macaulay somewhere says, that it is extraordinary that, whereas the laws of the motions of the heavenly bodies, far removed as they are from us, are perfectly well understood, the laws of the human mind, which are under our observation all day and every day, are no better understood than they were two thousand years ago.

But how much more extraordinary is it that, whereas what we might call the coxcombries of education—*e.g.*, the elements of astronomy—are now taught to every school-girl, neither mothers of families of any class, nor school-mistresses of any class, nor nurses of children, nor nurses of hospitals, are taught anything about those laws which God has assigned to the relations of our bodies with the world in which He has put them. In other words, the laws which make these bodies, into which He has put our minds, healthy or unhealthy organs of those minds, are all but unlearnt. Not but that these laws—the laws of life—are in a certain measure understood, but not even mothers think it worth their while to study them—to study how to give their children healthy existences. They call it medical or physiological knowledge, fit only for doctors.

ANOTHER OBJECTION.

We are constantly told,—"But the circumstances which govern our children's healths are beyond our control. What can we do with winds? There is the east wind. Most people can tell before they get up in the morning whether the wind is in the east."

To this one can answer with more certainty than to the former objections. Who is it who knows when the wind is in the east? Not the Highland drover, certainly, exposed to the east wind, but the young lady who is worn out with the want of exposure to fresh air, to sunlight, &c. Put the latter under as good sanitary circumstances as the former, and she too will not know when the wind is in the east.

AN CHAPTER FROM
Notes on Nursing, 1860

Printed in Great Britain
by Amazon

19921738R00130